LESION ANALYSIS IN NEUROPSYCHOLOGY

LESION ANALYSIS IN

NEUROPSYCHOLOGY

HANNA DAMASIO

ANTONIO R. DAMASIO

Department of Neurology
University of Iowa College of Medicine

New York   Oxford
OXFORD UNIVERSITY PRESS
1989

Oxford University Press

Oxford   New York   Toronto
Delhi   Bombay   Calcutta   Madras   Karachi
Petaling Jaya   Singapore   Hong Kong   Tokyo
Nairobi   Dar es Salaam   Cape Town
Melbourne   Auckland

and associated companies in
Berlin   Ibadan

Published by Oxford University Press, Inc.,
200 Madison Avenue, New York, New York 10016

Oxford is a registered trademark of Oxford University Press

Library of Congress Cataloging-in-Publication Data
Damasio, Hanna.
Lesion analysis in neuropsychology / Hanna Damasio, Antonio R. Damasio.
p.   cm.
Includes bibliographies and index.
ISBN 0-19-503919-X
1. Brain—Imaging.   2. Neuropsychiatry—Technique.   3. Brain—Anatomy.
4. Brain—Diseases—Diagnosis.   5. Tomography.
6. Magnetic resonance imaging.   I. Damasio, Antonio R.   II. Title.
[DNLM: 1. Brain—physiopathology.   2. Diagnostic Imaging.
3. Nervous System—anatomy & histology.   4. Neuropsychology.   WL 101 D171a]
RC473.B7D36   1989
616.8′04757—dc19
DNLM/DLC   for Library of Congress   88-39570   CPI (Rev.)

9 8 7 6 5 4 3 2

Printed in the United States of America
on acid-free paper

TO NORMAN GESCHWIND

ACKNOWLEDGMENTS

Although all the material used in this volume was personally studied over a period of 12 years, we must thank numerous colleagues who contributed generously to this research effort. In particular, we would like to acknowledge the support of colleagues in the Department of Radiology, who made sure the quality of the images on which our neuroanatomical studies are based was excellent. They are Steven Cornell, MD, Chief of the Neuroradiology section; Peter T. Kirchner, MD, Director of the Division of Nuclear Medicine Chief of the PET facility; Karim Rezai, MD, also of the Division of Nuclear Medicine; and William Yuh, MD, and James Ehrhardt, PhD, who are in charge of the MRI facility. We would also like to acknowledge a long-lasting collaboration with our colleagues in the Division of Cerebrovascular Diseases (Department of Neurology), under the direction of Harold P. Adams, MD.

We are grateful to our associate, Daniel Tranel, PhD, Director of the Benton Neuropsychology Laboratory at the Division of Behavioral Neurology and Cognitive Neuroscience, for his continued support and encouragement.

Arthur L. Benton, PhD, and Gary W. Van Hoesen, PhD, provided valuable critical advice at numerous points in the development of this project.

Paul Eslinger, PhD; Neill Graff-Radford, MD; Matthew Rizzo, MD; Steven Anderson, PHD; and Robert Dallas Jones, PhD; called our attention to many interesting cases and discussed several aspects of our methodology and findings.

The photographic material owes its quality to the outstanding technical competence and dedication of Paul C. Reimann.

Jon Spradling helped coordinate materials for the volume, with his unfailing attention to detail. Betty Redeker prepared the manuscript with her usual patience and good humor.

CONTENTS

LESION ANALYSIS IN NEUROPSYCHOLOGY

1
INTRODUCTION

The advent of computerized X-ray tomography (CT) and magnetic resonance scanning (MR) has revolutionized the use of the lesion method in humans by permitting the anatomical definition of focal brain lesions in living subjects. The general purpose of this volume is to discuss some means to cope with the many methodological problems posed by these technologies. Specifically, it describes a set of procedures that can be used to obtain the best possible neuroanatomical information from brain images. Although the focus is on the methodology that can make lesion studies possible, we also attempted, with our choice of examples throughout the volume, to illustrate advances in knowledge resulting from the use of the lesion method in humans. To achieve this, both text and the figure captions contain important information on the patients' neuropsychological profile. As a whole, the collection of illustrations constitutes an atlas of neuropsychological disorders seen from the vantage point of their neuroanatomical correlates. For this reason, we have included a thematic index to assist in the search of important exemplars of aphasia, agnosia, amnesia, and others.

The book opens with an overview of the lesion method as it can currently be applied to humans in the study of neuropsychological disorders, and with a brief review of some of the recent contributions the lesion method has made to the understanding of the neural substrates of mental processes. A new model of the neural substrates of cognition inspired by results obtained with the method completes the opening section.

The reader should know about the sources of the material used here. All of the examples in this volume come from our own studies of the neuroanatomical correlates of neuropsychological disorders carried out in the Division of Behavioral Neurology and Cognitive Neuroscience of the University of Iowa. By design, the anatomical study of all imaging material is systematically carried out, in independent fashion, by investigators blind to the subjects' neuropsychological status and with no knowledge whatever of the cognitive experiments in which they are involved or of the results thereof. This unusual approach, aimed at reducing investigator bias in the collection of anatomical data, calls for the masking of all identification information on each subject's film transparencies and for a filing code on the basis of which information can be stored.

The subjects whose images come under analysis are entered into our projects by yet another group of independent investigators according to dual criteria: (a) presence of a focal lesion anywhere in the cerebrum, regardless of whether or not there is an accompanying neuropsychological disorder, or (b) presence of a neuropsychological disorder regardless of whether or not a structural lesion has been detected. The aim is again to reduce sample biasing through the use of anatomical or psychological selection criteria as much as that is reasonable, and to permit the manifestation of false positive or false negative results as far as anatomical/cognitive correlations are concerned.

All subjects entered into our projects are studied with a core neuropsychological battery that screens for the presence of major cognitive defects in the areas of perception, memory, language, thought processes, problem-solving abilities, and personality. Depending on the type of neuropsychological disturbance identified in the core study, the subjects are then recruited into special projects and studied with specific sets of neuropsychological tests. In a final phase, experiments motivated by a variety of hypotheses under scrutiny are undertaken.

The reconciliation of anatomical and cognitive data takes place at different levels and under different circumstances. For instance, regular meetings occur, during which the blind codes are opened and cases are reviewed. Also, as studies focused on a given topic are undertaken, further in-depth analysis of anatomical/cognitive correlations takes place.

The ultimate goal behind this design is to generate substantial samples of comparable natural lesions so that the associations that may be established between lesions and abnormal behaviors at a single case-study level can be credibly replicated. In brief, the aim is to minimize the consequences of the vagaries of human neuropathology and to approximate, in the human cognitive neuroscience laboratory the control conditions available to the experimental neuropsychologist who works with animals. The substantial groups of

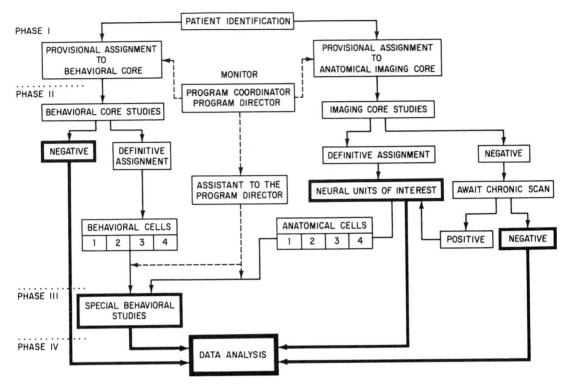

CHART 1.1. Flow chart depicting the parallel and independent routes for data collection and analysis of experimental subjects at our laboratories. The behavioral/cognitive route is in the left column, and the neuroanatomical one in the right.

patients with similar lesions that we have been able to form over the years certainly dispel the myth that lesion studies in humans are fatally flawed by the impossibility of replicating the anatomical and neuropsychologic characteristics of any single case. Both the possibility of replication and the possibility of controlling the specificity of an effect are available with human studies. For obvious reasons, and even after the best of efforts, it is not possible to achieve full experimental control in the human setting. But neither is it possible for the animal experimenter to have available subjects with a cognitive architecture similar to that of humans.

Because the focus of this work is neuroanatomy, as viewed through neuroimaging techniques, the illustrations and their accompanying legends comprise the core of the volume. A word about the conventions used in the illustrations is in order. The CT, MR, and Single Photon Emission Tomography (SPET) images depicted in each illustration are always oriented in the following way:

1. With transverse or axial cuts, the left hemisphere appears on the left-hand side and the right hemisphere on the right; the sequence of cuts is always from lower to higher.

2. With coronal cuts, the sides are reversed, that is, the left hemisphere appears on the right and the right hemisphere on the left; the sequence of cuts is from anterior to posterior, that is, anterior cuts are shown first.

The problems faced by researchers using neuroimaging material as a basis for their lesion studies are discussed in Chapter 3. A specific method of neuroanatomical analysis applicable to CT and MR images is described in Chapter 4. An Appendix includes the several sets of anatomical templates necessary to implement the procedures described in Chapter 4.

2
THE LESION METHOD
IN HUMANS

Overview

The essence of the lesion method is the establishment of a correlation between a circumscribed region of damaged brain and changes in some aspect of an experimentally controlled behavioral performance. Given a preexisting theory about the operation of the normal brain and how it would mediate the performance of an experimental task, the lesion (the area of brain damage) can be seen as a probe to test the validity of the theories, that is, a means to decide if the account of brain organization and operation provided by a given model is or is not falsifiable.

The lesion method has a broad scope of application. The subjects may be human or animal. The lesion may have been produced by neurological disease or by a surgical procedure, may be small or large, and may be studied *in-vivo* or *post-mortem*. The prime requirement is that it be confined and referable to some specifiable neuroanatomical unit. The measure of postlesion changes can be made on the basis of within subject baseline observations or on the basis of comparisons across control subjects. In this volume, we deal only with human lesions, produced by neurological disease or surgical ablation, and studied *in vivo* with modern neuroimaging techniques.

The lesion method has a long history dating back at least to Morgagni's classic demonstrations of the association between unilateral brain disease and sensory and motor disabilities on the opposite side of the body. Bouillaud's (1825) attempt to link post-mortem findings of frontal lobe lesions to the occurrence of speech disorders during life represented the first major correlational study of psychology and anatomy. In the 1860s, Broca's correlation of aphasia with focal damage to the left frontal lobe initiated the modern era of lesional localization of neuropsychological disabilities.

The latter decades of the nineteenth century witnessed an enthusiastic and vigorous application of the lesion method, an application that was responsible for some path-breaking discoveries, as well as for the development of a new approach to the understanding of brain function. However, although the findings were generally replicated and gained wide acceptance, the theories that were advanced in connection with the findings met with considerable resistance.

As best exemplified by the aphasiologists Wernicke (1874) and Lichtheim (1885), pioneering neurologists conceived of the existence of brain "centers" capable of performing a variety of complex psychological functions with relative independence. What little interaction there was among those few, noncontiguous centers was achieved by unidirectional nerve bundles or pathways. These strikingly novel but simple concepts were subject to deserved criticisms, perhaps the most penetrating of which came from Sigmund Freud, in the days that preceded his psychoanalytic theorization (Freud, 1891) and from Hughlings Jackson (1866–1891). Quite understandably, by the early part of this century, the theoretical account had lost favor and influence, incompatible as it was with the more detailed knowledge of neurology and psychology that had later become available. Unfortunately, because the lesion method was closely interwoven with the theory, the method followed its inventors' fortunes. Indirectly, the theory's downfall contributed to a relative neglect of the lesion method as a valid means of scientific inquiry, an explainable but regrettable loss.

The lesion method once again attained prominence in the 1960s. In part, this development was a reaction to the excesses of "equipotential" antilocalizationism, as well as to the impasse generated by "black-box" behaviorism. However, this revival, powerfully supported by Geschwind's (1965) innovative thinking, also reflected the conviction that the lesion method was a principal means to investigate the neural basis of human behavior and cognition. The realization that this was so emerged gradually from the work of several neuropsychologists, among whom the most prominent were A. R. Luria, Henri Hécaen, Brenda Milner, Arthur Benton, Hans-Lukas Teuber, and Oliver Zangwill. Curiously, the rehabilitation of the lesion method began more than a decade ahead of the then unforeseeable development of the finer neuroimaging technologies that would solidly reinstate this approach—computerized X-ray tomography only had its inception in 1973, and only became a viable neuropsychological method by the late 1970s. Magnetic resonance scanning (MR) emerged in the early 1980s.

Also, it is gradually becoming evident that the lesion method should be separated from the theoretical accounts that are based on findings obtained through its agency. As is the case with any other approach, the lesion method has its limitations and misapplications. The validity of the method is not an issue. The lesion method is one entity, with its inherent virtues and pitfalls. The theoretical constructs that make use of the lesion method are another. When improperly used, the lesion method can lead to invalid data and misleading interpretations, a shortcoming it shares with any methodology. But nothing prevents practitioners of the lesion method from proposing the richest and most dynamic accounts of brain function.

It is startling to see theoretical inadequacies blamed on the use of the lesion method itself rather than on the conceptualization that attempted to account for findings it helped generate, as if data collected by this approach would irrevocably have led investigators to conceive nothing but discrete processing centers, or would have bound innocent investigators to "diagram-maker" centers, "single-purpose" pathways, or "grandmother" neurons. This is simply not so.

Naturally, the lesion method can only be as good as the finest level of cognitive characterization and anatomical resolution it uses. In other words, the method's yield is limited by:

1. The sophistication of the neuropsychological testing or experimentation with which anatomical lesions are correlated;
2. The sophistication of the theoretical constructs and hypotheses being tested by the lesion probes;
3. The degree of sophistication with which the nervous tissue is conceptualized, that is, how the missing processing units are viewed anatomically and physiologically, the type of network from which they are missing, the level at which those neurally defined networks establish contact with some level of cognitive architecture;
4. The anatomical resolution of the procedures used.

It is clear that until quite recently, because of technical limitations, several of these methodological features have been weak. For example, cognitive structures have not been teased apart, componentially, but rather have been considered as a conflated unit. The gross amalgamation commonly referred to as "auditory comprehension" in the study of acquired language disorders is as good an example as any of how numerous cognitively separable structures and processes have been conceptualized as unitary and measured as one.

As far as work in humans is concerned, the current progress in the lesion method is due to: (a) advances in the conceptualization of brain tissue, with the ensuing progress in the theoretical accounts of neural operation; (b) advances in theoretical formulations of cognitive processes and development of experimental neuropsychological probes; and (c) technological advances that have resulted in the ensuing refinement of neuroimaging definition.

All of these advances have contributed substantially to the empirical efficacy of the lesion method. The conceptual and technological advances in neuropsychological and neuroimaging investigation, respectively, have decreased the error variance associated with brain-behavior experimentation, increased the sensitivity of the lesion method, and allowed for more fine-grained specifications at the theoretical level. The latter, in turn, have led to a greater degree of precision in the formulation of hypotheses and boosted the statistical power of experiments that more often than not must rely on small subject groups or even single cases. Improved reliability, on both the neuropsychological and neuroimaging sides of the equation, has increased the validity of the lesion method.

New Concepts Regarding
Brain Tissue Structure and Function

Leaving aside developments in subcellular neurobiology, which do not have a direct bearing on the lesion method, the past two decades brought some major changes to the conceptualization of brain tissue organization and function.

The columnar and laminar organization of the cerebral cortex and the intricate patterns of neural projections interconnecting cortical and noncortical regions are now far better understood (see Jones & Peters, 1986).

To the idea of center contained within a grossly defined cortical gyrus, had succeeded the notion of cytoarchitectonic area, defined in histological terms and on the basis of neuron types and laminar arrangement [Figure 2.1]. At first, such areas appeared to subtend a relatively unified role, for example, the primary sensory and motor cortices. But currently, cytoarchitectonic areas, especially in association cortices, have yielded smaller functional subregions within themselves. These are defined on the basis of the electrophysiological behavior of single neurons or neuronal populations as they respond to specific types of stimuli or their properties, alone or in combination, or as they are engaged in various forms of motor response (Allman, Miezin, & McGuiness, 1985; Mountcastle, Lynch, & Georgopoulos, 1975; Van Essen & Maunsell, 1983; Zeki, 1977). The visual system is the standard example of this new parcellation, illustrated in Figure 2.2. Even the primary sensory cortices have yielded to parcellation, with different neuron columns being differentially dedicated to different stimuli properties. (Livingstone & Hubel, 1984) [See Figure 2.3]

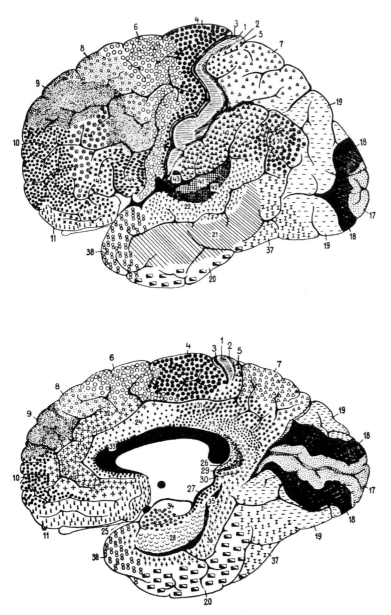

FIGURE 2.1. Lateral and mesial view of a human brain with the cytoarchitectonic areas proposed by Brodmann in 1909. Although it is now clear that cytoarchitectonic areas are not "centers" for complex psychological functions, the breakdown of cortical tissue on the basis of cytoarchitecture remains critical as a reference for anatomical and physiological studies. Neuroanatomists agree that Brodmann not only made a major scientific contribution but did so with as few errors as one can reasonably expect.

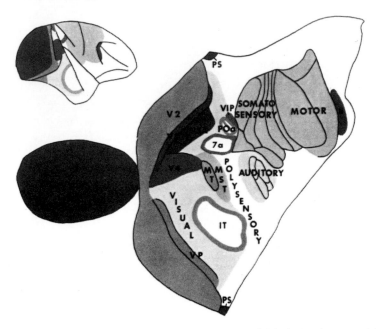

FIGURE 2.2. Functional subregions of a monkey's unfolded visual cortex. Most of the many fields depicted here are the offspring of the classical visual areas 17, 18, and 19. (Reproduced with permission from Van Essen & Maunsell, *Trends in Neurosciences* **63**:370–377, 1983).

Depending on the type of cortex, the connections encountered in adult brains are established in divergent or convergent manner, either on the principle of one-to-many or one-to-few, but always from one unit to a limited set. (The issue of those connections' development, with its complex phenomena of neuronal death and competition of surviving neurons, is beyond the scope of this chapter; see Cowan, 1973; Cowan et al, 1984; Purves & Lichtman, 1980; and Rakic, 1979, 1985, for review). In general, primary sensory cortices signal widely to a set of functional regions within the encircling "early" association cortices, in a strongly parallel fashion. Subregions of those cortices project to several higher-order cortices. Feedback pathways reciprocate those projections to their points of origin and also to other cortical points. Signals can thus lead to *retro*activation in multiple feeding sites, as well as to activation in numerous other sites, upstream, downstream, or at the same level of the network, depending on the dynamic firing patterns the network will generate. In brief, brain tissue contains numerous systems, composed of networks that are made up of functional regions interconnected by feed-forward and feedback projections. Those systems' operation is best described by the attributes parallel, serial, recursive, and nonlinear (see third section of this chapter; also A. Damasio, 1989 a and b; A. Damasio, H. Damasio, & Tranel, 1989).

The kind of information that constitutes memory's raw contents is seen as stored in the cerebral cortices, but in ensembles of interconnected neuronal columns rather than in single neurons, that is, in distributed fashion. Likewise, complex psychological activities are not viewed as the result of the operation of a single area or even a single functional region, but rather as the consequence of concerted activity in networks made up of multiple regions. Intriguingly, this new outlook moves away from both the neurological concepts of the nineteenth century, influenced as they were by phrenology, and from the antilocalizationist component of Lashley's ideas that held sway in our century until the 1950s, according to which all association cortices were functionally equipotential and virtually interchangeable (Lashley, 1950). From this vantage point, the traditional "local-

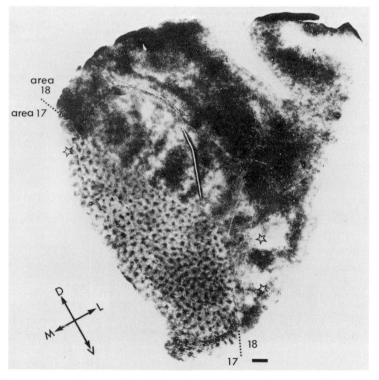

FIGURE 2.3. Cortex of areas 17 and 18 stained with cytochrome oxidase. The mottled sectors of area 17 ("blobs") correspond to cell columns dedicated to color processing. Interspersed cell columns are more involved with the processing of several aspects of form. The "stripes" of the adjoining area 18 are also functionally separate. (Reproduced with permission from Livingstone & Hubel, *Journal of Neuroscience* **4**:309–356, 1984).

ization" of psychological activities is both a misconceived and unattainable goal. By contrast, a feasible and legitimate aim appears to be the identification of neural systems related to certain types of cognitive operation, and the probing of putative networks involved in components of such operations.

From Behaviorism to Cognitive Science

The changes on the mind side of the equation have also been pronounced. The most salient was the shift away from the behaviorist model of psychology, which had made the relationship between stimuli and response the only legitimate object of study and treated mind and brain alike as a black box. In its place, a cognitive model that reinstates the reality of mental phenomena and makes nonverbal as well as verbal representations a valid focus of psychological inquiry has gained acceptance. The work of Posner (1980), Triesman (Triesman & Gelade, 1980), Kosslyn (1980), and Shepard (Shepard & Cooper, 1982) on the processes of attention and visual imagery in normal individuals illustrates the change. In the new approach, subjects' behavioral responses are not just linked to the stimuli that eventually triggered them, but are connected to mind processes and representations that handled the stimulus and generated the responses according to some mechanism. The investigators no longer shy away from formulating hypotheses about those mechanisms and attempting to test their validity, indirectly, by measuring external responses.

The past three decades have witnessed a notable development of high diverse theories and methodologies that are loosely bound together by their focus on the phenomena of the mind. Linguistics and psycholinguistics, numerous brands of cognitive psychology, traditional artificial intelligence, along with the newer computational modeling approaches to psychological processes, are all part of this broad and still evolving field, which can be designated *cognitive science* for lack of a better name. For some, the scope and historical meaning of this development constitute a true revolution (Gardner, 1985). In the very least, even broadly defined, it is apparent that the cognitive sciences offer the possibility of eventually achieving a true biology of the mind.

Advances in Neuropsychological Techniques and Experimental Design

No less important than these theoretical developments were advances in the armamentarium of available neuropsychological techniques. First, throughout the 1970s and 1980s, several classical neuropsychological instruments have become standard. This is certainly the case with many tests in the aphasia batteries of Goodglass and Kaplan, Benton, and Kertesz, and with several tests of nonverbal processing (see Benton et al, 1983; Goodglass & Kaplan, 1972; Kertesz, 1979; and Lezak, 1983). In addition, numerous experimental techniques originating with the fields of psycholinguistics, psychophysics, psychophysiology, and cognitive psychology, in general, have been applied with success to the work with brain-damaged individuals. With such a variety of techniques available, a comprehensive list would not be possible here. The following is a brief list of studies that provide a sample of their application: Bellugi, Poizner and Klima, 1983; Blumstein, 1978; Bradley, Garret, & Zurif, 1980; Caplan & Futter, 1986; Caramazza & Zurif, 1976; Farah, 1989; Fromkin, 1987; Gardner et al, 1983; Kean, 1977; Marshall & Newcombe, 1973; Rizzo & H. Damasio, 1985; Rizzo, Hurtig, & A. Damasio, 1987; Saffran, Schwartz, & Marin, 1980; Schwartz, Marin, & Saffran, 1980; Tranel & A. Damasio, 1985.

An important issue of experimental design has also been brought to the fore in recent years. It relates to the use of single cases versus groups of cases in neuropsychological research and it clearly is of special import in studies that overtly or implicitly claim to use the lesion method. Our position is that both single-case studies and group studies can be valid, but little doubt exists that few centers of neuropsychological investigation have available the range of techniques and the large number of human lesion cases necessary to satisfy the research requirements of group studies. Furthermore, we view the ideal approach as the collection of and reflection on *multiple single-case studies.* In our center, such cases are fully characterized neuroanatomically, and the neuroanatomical definition is used as an independent variable. The controls for each subject are other subjects whose lesions overlap with, or abut, the boundaries of the target subject's lesion. In a way, such collections of single-case studies constitute groups too, but they share little with the traditional aggregation of cases on the basis of neuropsychological syndromes or symptoms, or even on the basis of the presence or absence of lesions in a broadly defined brain region: "anterior versus posterior," "quadrants," "lobes," "hemispheres." Our ultimate goal is the link of neuropsychological features and dimensions, to specific lesion probes, on the basis of theoretically motivated accounts of neural/cognitive relationships. Naturally, as the number of in-depth multiple, single studies grows, there also grows the possibility of comparing neuropsychological profiles of individuals contrasted on the basis of anatomical differences.

Another pertinent methodological issue relates to the neuropsychological taxonomies. Although none of our current research is based on any syndromatic classification of the classical neuropsychological disorders, clearly, communication among clinicians and researchers must rely, for the foreseeable future, on the use of numerous convenient syndrome and symptom designations. However, whenever we use those terms, it should not be taken to mean that we subscribe, necessarily, to either the full classificatory validity of those entities, or to the neuropsychological and neurophysiological accounts that have been traditionally attached to them. In fact, we have reservations on both counts. The reasons are as follows.

As is the case with any taxonomic entity in medicine, clinical syndromes are characterized by a cluster of co-occurring signs that signifies the presence of a given disease process. In each instance of classification, the cluster may be surrounded by a varied degree of additional signs or by none at all. There need not be any causal relation among the signs, mere coincidence being sufficient. A syndrome's clinical validity is measurable by the accuracy of the predictions it generates.

In neurology, and especially in the neurology of cognition, the syndrome is used to predict a lesion location rather than a disease process, and its validity is thus checked in relation to an anatomical prediction, rather than a prediction of pathological process. This poses problems because numerous forms of pathology can affect the same location, with different consequences. Another problem derives from the design and workings of the nervous system in relation to cognition: the distributiveness and relative redundancy of functions within and across anatomical networks is such that similar, albeit not precisely equal, syndromes can result from dysfunction in different neural sites. Consequently, when factors such as individual biological and educational variables are added, the accuracy of syndrome-based predictions can be reduced. We believe that, provided expert judgment is exercised, syndromes remain extremely useful tools for clinicians. However, given the situation described previously, their use as sole predictors of anatomical lesions in research projects is hardly acceptable.

Localization of Damage and the Nonlocalizability of Complex Psychological Functions

The classically discovered links between certain regions of the cerebral cortex and signs of neuropsychological disorder have been thoroughly validated, remain a staple of clinical neurology, and permit relatively accurate cerebral *localization of damage,* that is, more often than not the presence of certain neuropsychological defects indicates to the clinical expert that dysfunction is present in a specific brain area, information that may be put to good use in the patient's clinical management. However, these links do not authorize cerebral *localization of function,* that is, they do not mean that a function disturbed by the lesion was somehow inscribed in the tissue destroyed by the lesion.

The distinction between the possible and accurate localizability of damage, given psychological defects, and the nonlocalizability of complex psychological functions is critical. It is important to realize that clinical knowledge of localization is valid, useful, *and* compatible with the rejection of simplistic physiological interpretations based on such knowledge.

That cortical centers, as traditionally conceived, could not form the basis for the complex psychological functions studied in neuropsychology has long been apparent. But the neural architecture revealed by neuroanatomy and neurophysiology, along with the cognitive architecture revealed by experimental neuropsychology and linguistics, have made it clear that single-center functions, single-purpose pathways, or unidirectional cascades of information process are simply inconceivable. Furthermore, mere reflection on the residual performance that follows focal brain insults, as well as the ensuing patterns of recovery, calls for types of neural organization in which knowledge must, of necessity, be widely distributed at multiple neural levels, and complex psychological functions must emerge from the cooperation of multiple components of integrated networks (see third section of this chapter).

Perhaps the lesion method's greatest intrinsic limitation resides with its reliance on conceiving "normal function" on the basis of the subtraction of a given set of inoperative processing units from a network, rather than on the basis of the regular working of those units. Indeed, major risks exist in the intellectual exercise necessary to conceptualize normal structure and function from damaged structure and deviant function, and the danger can only be reduced by the quality of the theoretical framework and of the tight formulation of hypotheses under scrutiny.

However, lesions can certainly be used as probes to the operation of hypothetical networks of anatomical regions designed to perform a specified function cooperatively. Given the basic characteristics of the network—in terms of the constitution of its units and their connectional arrangement—lesion probes in different points of the network can help define the cooperative role of the diverse units based on contrasts of the behavioral performances linked to different sites of damage. The method's power is limited by the lesions' size and by the richness of the "psychological" operations hypothesized for the network the lesion is probing. The smaller the lesion probe capable of creating discriminatory effects (that is, the smaller the lesion capable of causing a functional perturbation that can be related unequivocally to a certain sector of the network), the more the lesion method will have to contribute.

The Lesion Method and
the Dynamic Varieties of Brain Mapping

Partly overlapping with the extraordinary development of CT and MR, emission tomography (ET) is now coming of age. The method stems from earlier studies of regional cerebral blood flow that measured the washout of radionuclides from the brain as detected by lateral skull probes. In essence, it combines the principle that regional distribution of a radio-labeled substance can serve as an index to local neural activity with the tomographic reconstruction techniques that permit detailed neuroanatomical reconstructions. Whether using single photons (as in single photon emission tomography, or SPET), or positrons (positron emission tomography, or PET), several research centers are now equipped to perform this type of study using a large array of radioactive isotopes and obtaining varied degrees of neuropsychological resolution.

The technical problems posed by ET and the numerous methodological issues it raises have been stumbling blocks and are far from solved. The resolution remains limited and the anatomical localization procedures are not as reliable as those that have been developed for static imaging. The major issue, however, is that the regional activity changes that the best of these techniques can detect, are likely to result from superimpositions of activity in functional nets that represent concurrent but not necessarily related operations in overlapping systems and networks. In other words, increase or decrease of radiosignal in a given region can not be equated, for certain, with the putative operation of a hypothesized unit of a cognitive network. It is clear, however, that major progress is ahead and critical new data about brain function will eventually come from those techniques.

ET offers not only a somewhat more direct functional index of neural activity but permits, in addition, the study of some neural correlates of cognitive activity in *normal* individuals. This frees the method from a major constraint of the lesion method, which is the necessary reliance on individuals with focal brain lesions. It is important to note that ET is an addition to the so-called "static" forms of imaging and not a superseding alternative. In fact, ET and the lesion method can go together in many ways. ET can be used in subjects with lesions, in which case it becomes a useful complement to the static lesion studies obtained with CT and MR. Even the finest form of dynamic imaging conceivable in the foreseeable future is not a solution for the theoretical problems posed by the attempt to map a cognitive organization on a neural one, or vice-versa. It is just another welcome avenue of information gathering.

Another powerful method of dynamic brain mapping is the study of electrical brain stimulation in patients about to undergo surgery for the treatment of epilepsy, an approach best exemplified by the current work of Ojemann (1983). The comments made about ET can be applied here as well. These methods should not be seen as superseding the lesion method. They can be used to test, at least in part, hypotheses formulated on the basis of the lesion method, and the information they yield can be tested, at least in part, by the lesion method. They are fully compatible and welcome additions to the methodological stock of cognitive neuroscience.

The advent of neuroimaging technologies capable of fine lesion detection and neuroanatomical resolution has entirely revolutionized the lesion method's application in humans and has already led to critical advances in the understanding of the anatomical substrates of cognition.

The Issues of Material and Technique

In many respects, studies based on post-mortem material provide the desirable standard for the lesion method. The anatomical description of the lesion at macroscopic level can be fairly complete, and the histological study of the surrounding tissue may provide information about the damage's real boundary. Under optimal conditions of tissue collection, it may even be possible to study the impairment of projections related to the damaged area (A. Damasio & Van Hoesen, 1979; Mesulam, 1979). However, autopsy material poses major problems. One is that the time of autopsy does not generally coincide with the epoch of clinical observation and experimental study. Frequently, several years intervene between one and the other, which is an obstacle to valid correlations between altered neuroanatomy and cognitive state. Another problem, of a practical nature, is the rarity of autopsy material among the victims of stroke or herpes simplex encephalitis, the two conditions that, as will be explained in Chapter 3, constitute the most desirable targets for lesion research. The number of post-mortem studies pertinent to the study of cognition were always few, even in the nineteenth century, and medical progress has simply made that number dwindle to the point that systematic study of groups of subjects is virtually impossible.

Under certain circumstances, autopsy material may be the only way to gain insight into the nervous system's disordered structure, in which case the undesirable lack of temporal correlation between neuropsychological and anatomical observations must be overlooked. For instance, the study of the cellular and laminar distribution of neurofibrillary tangles in post-mortem tissue from patients with Alzheimer's disease has revealed a pattern that no study performed in experimental animals or in humans with *in vivo* neuroimaging methods would have predicted or shown [see Figure 2.4].

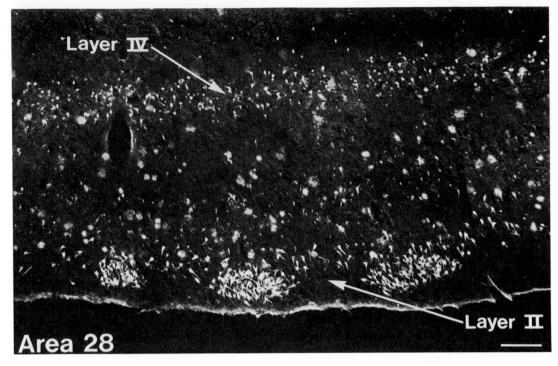

FIGURE 2.4. Section of entorhinal cortex from the brain of a patient with Alzheimer's disease. (The entorhinal cortex is located in the mesial and anterior aspect of the temporal lobe, within the parahippocampal gyrus, or fifth temporal gyrus.) The arrows point to Layers II and IV of this critical cortex. The white stained cells correspond to neurofibrillary tangles marked by Congo red. Note that the tangles form clusters in Layer II, are virtually absent in Layer III, and are again frequent in Layer IV. This image is representative of the distribution of cellular pathology in Alzheimer's patients. The selectivity of the damage is remarkable and accomplishes a complete disconnection of the hippocampus. This is because Layer II of the entorhinal cortex is the point of emergence of the perforant pathway, the principal source of input to the hippocampus, whereas Layer IV is the principal source of output from the hippocampus back to the cerebral cortex.

Some Fundamental Discoveries Based on the Lesion Method and Their Theoretical Consequences

Findings obtained with the lesion method are currently having a major impact on the understanding of the neural basis of perception, memory, and language. These new discoveries not only expand knowledge regarding the neural basis, of cognition but virtually demand the adoption of new theoretical models to account for higher function (see third section of this chapter, and A. Damasio, 1989 a and b, for an example of such a model).

Perception

Of the developments related to perception, discoveries in the domain of vision dominate the field, as they also do where other methodologies are concerned. Lesion studies confirm unequivocally that not only are the left and right visual systems functionally asymmetric, as implied in the work of Sperry and collaborators (Sperry, 1961), but also that the inferior and superior components of the visual system are functionally different. Furthermore, they imply that there is a considerable degree of additional functional segregation, according to which different regions within the broader sectors of the system are especially dedicated to particular types of processing such as color, or form, or motion. Finally, to make matters more complicated, there is also evidence that, notwithstanding marked channel segregation, the specialized subregions interact among themselves intricately to produce the sort of integrated perceptual processes humans are capable of experiencing.

In general, the system's inferior or ventral component, on either side, appears to be devoted more to the processing of some of the

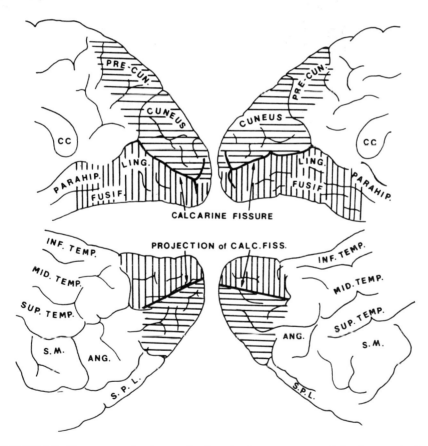

FIGURE 2.5. The supracalcarine and infracalcarine territories of the human brain. In the mesial aspect, the distinction is easily made by the calcarine fissure. In the lateral aspect, the distinction is made by the imaginary prolongation of a horizontal plane set at the average orientation and incidence of the calcarine fissures. Note the marked asymmetry of these regions.

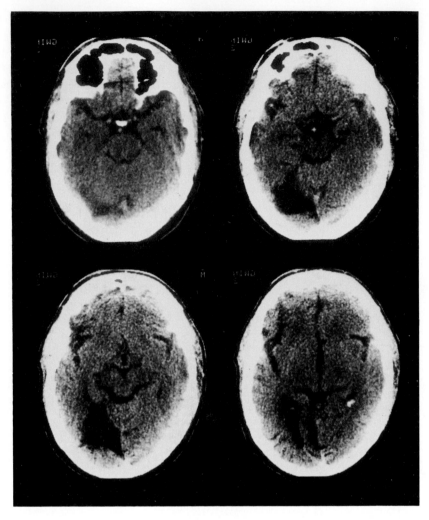

(A)

FIGURE 2.6. CT (A) and corresponding templates (B) of a 67-year-old, right-handed man, obtained 16 months after he suddenly developed loss of vision in the right visual field. Evaluation of visual loss revealed a complete right superior quadrantanopia but normal form vision in the lower right quadrant, where he was unable to see color. Within that quadrant, objects were seen in shades of gray; that is, he had a right inferior quadrant achromatopsia. He was alexic, but writing was normal. Sixteen months later, at the time CT was obtained, his reading ability had improved, although reading speed was still below premorbid level. The right superior quadrantanopia and the right inferior achromatopsia remained unchanged. (For an example of complete left hemiachromatopsia without any defect in form vision, see A. Damasio et al, 1980. For an example of full-field achromatopsia, see Figure 2.8).

The combination of a quadrant form vision defect, with quadrant color loss, within the same half-field is not infrequent. It is the result of a re-

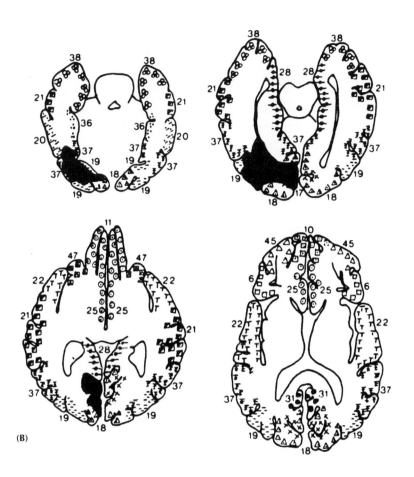

(B)

stricted lesion that damages only one sector of the form-processing cortices but destroys all or most of some key color-processing cortices. In other words, this patient would have had color loss in the entire right visual field (a right hemiachromatopsia), were it not for the form vision loss in the upper quadrant, which effectively precludes *any* vision.

The lesion in this case is in the infracalcarine association cortices of the left hemisphere. It extends anteriorly into the occipitotemporal junc-

tion and superiorly, on the mesial aspect, into the calcarine region. It is not possible, from these transverse cuts, to ascertain if it destroys the calcarine cortices. (Other incidences are needed to decide on this question; see Chapter 4).

Note that, as in all transverse brain images (CT and MR) the left hemisphere is on the left and the right on the right. Investigators in our group are now attempting to characterize achromatopsia in psychophysic terms.

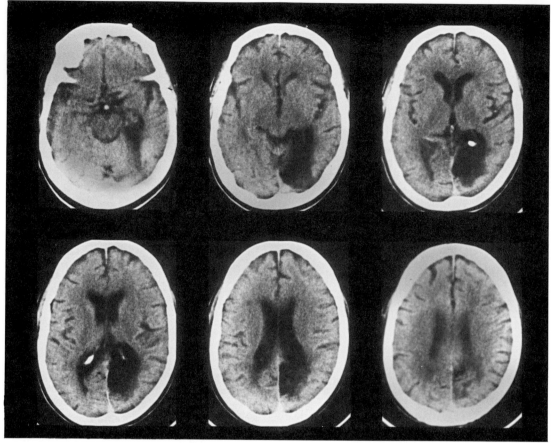

(A)

FIGURE 2.7. CT (A) and corresponding templates (B) of a 72-year-old, right-handed man who had the sudden onset of left hemianopia due to a large right occipital infarct. Color and form vision were intact in his right visual field. He had no difficulty in recognizing himself, his family, or his friends by vision alone; that is, he did not have prosopagnosia. He could read and write normally and had no language-processing defect. However, this patient had a severe defect of visual memory and visual learning, and had constructional apraxia.

The lesion in this case is in the infracalcarine

aspects of physical structure of the perceived entities, namely shape and color. The system's superior or dorsal component is more concerned with the spatial relationships among components of entities and with the placement of entities within a space. (As used here, the notion of *entity* covers virtually every stimulus in the environment, natural or man-made, animate or inanimate, small or large, and also applies to abstractions. Human faces, animals, manipulable instruments, vehicles, buildings, body parts, and so on, are all entities, their physical structure being defined by such *features* and *properties* as form at different scales, color, and movement. *Events* are the result of interplay among entities, in space and time.)

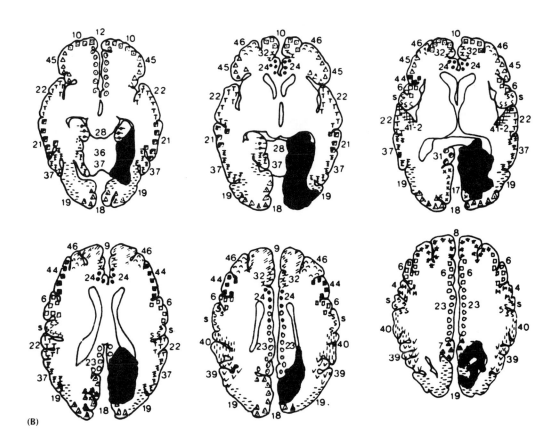

(B)

association cortices, but in the right hemisphere. It extends anteriorly into the occipitotemporal junction and into posterior hippocampal regions. In the mesial aspect, it extends higher than in the previous example, suggesting that it probably involves the supracalcarine region.

This patient does not show achromatopsia in the left visual field for the simple reason that the left field is blind; that is, hemianopia precludes the possibility of achromatopsia.

The visual association cortices located below the plane of the calcarine fissure (which contains area 17, or the primary visual cortex) are thus somewhat more concerned with the perception of entities themselves, that is, with *what* entities are, rather than with *where* they are relative to spatial coordinates or to other entities. [Figure 2.5]. It appears that most of the ventral cortices that process color and aspects of form do not process movement, although the exact position of the movement-related cortices in humans remains to be fully established. (The work of Zihl, Von Cramon, & Mai, 1983, as well as our own, suggests that lateral rather than mesial cortices are related to motion processing. From their position in humans, these

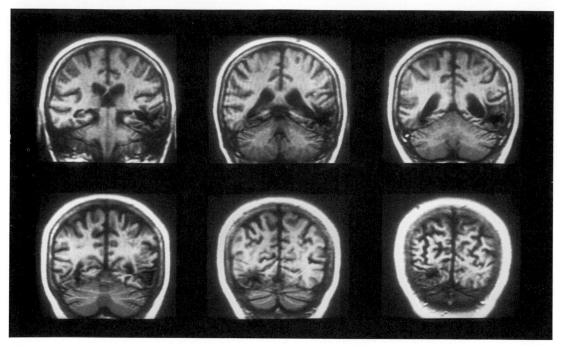

(A)

FIGURE 2.8. MR of a 67-year-old, right-handed woman who had sustained bilateral occipitotemporal infarcts six years earlier. (An earlier CT and cerebral blood flow image of the same patient appears in Figures 3.6 and 3.7.) Neuropsychological assessment of visual perception failed to reveal any defect. Stereopsis was normal and so was spatial contrast sensitivity. Yet, she was unable to recognize any previously familiar face, including her own. Nor could she learn to recognize the face of any of the people with whom she had come into contact after her stroke. She could, however, easily recognize friends and family from their voices. The condition is known as prosopagnosia. The patient's recognition defect extended to a variety of animate and inanimate objects, provided recognition of their specific identity was requested, and provided they were visually "ambiguous" (see A. Damasio et al, 1982b). This patient also had complete bilateral achromatopsia in the presence of almost intact fields for form vision (she had a small left peripheral superior quadrantic defect only).

cortices might actually stride the rigidly defined, dorsal and ventral components of the system, but the relative paucity of lesions circumscribed to the lateral occipital cortices has delayed understanding of this issue.)

These discoveries were based on the study of patients with circumscribed lesions confined to the subcalcarine portions of areas 18 and 19, who developed such conditions as hemiachromatopsia, alexia, prosopagnosia, and visual object agnosia (A. Damasio & H. Damasio, 1983; A. Damasio et al, 1980; A. Damasio, H. Damasio, & Van Hoesen, 1982b; Newcombe 1969; Meadows 1974a, 1974b) [see Figures 2.6 to 2.8, and 3.12].

The superior or dorsal visual association cortices, strictly speaking, the supracalcarine components of areas 18 and 19, are espe-

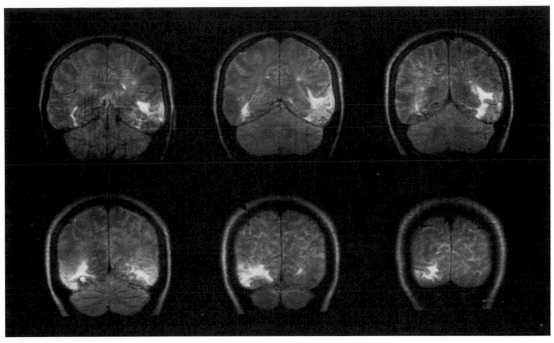

(B)

Both T_1 (A) and T_2 (B) weighted images show a bilateral lesion. The lesion in the left hemisphere (seen on the right side of each image) starts in the white matter of the inferior temporal regions (middle and inferior temporal gyri) and extends to the most posterior level of the occipital horn, where it involves infracalcarine association cortices. The lesion in the right hemisphere (seen on the left side of each image) starts more posteriorly, at the level of the mesial occipitotemporal junction and extends further back into the depth of the right occipital lobe, but always remains in infracalcarine region. The coronal cuts permit us to be certain about the lesion's position in relation to the calcarine region because the calcarine fissure is readily recognizable. These neuropsychological and neuroanatomical findings can be correlated with results of cognitive and psychophysiological experiments, in order to test hypothetical mechanisms of recognition.

cially concerned (a) with the spatial placement of entities within spaces, (b) with aspects of those entities' movements, and (c) with the assembly of an entity's components in an entity-intrinsic space. In this area, some original discoveries go back to the work of Gordon Holmes (1918 a & b), but recent work on patients with bilateral damage to these cortices confirm that they lose their ability to build a coherent image of their extra-personal space in such a way that the relationships among objects are no longer properly appreciated. The ability to attend to more than one object in clear vision is lost, and often there follows an inability to guide arm and hand movements properly towards objects in space (see A. Damasio, 1985a; Newcombe Ratcliff, 1989, for review) [see Figures 2.9 and 2.10].

A large literature related to these developments has dealt with other aspects of the disorders of visual spatial processing, including the phenomenon of neglect (see De Renzi, 1982; Heilman, Watson, & Valenstein, 1985; Mesulam, 1981; Newcombe & Ratcliff, 1989). The pertinent point in this context is that such work not only confirms the previously identified left–right functional asymmetry of the visual system, but suggests that a powerful ventral–dorsal dichotomy is also prevalent.

Stereovision is another ability whose neural substrate may be skewed towards the superior visual cortices (Rizzo & Damasio, 1985) and, as noted previously, evidence exists to suggest that some aspects of motion detection may also be anatomically linked to the dorsal sector.

These discoveries in humans parallel those made in nonhuman primates, using both the lesion method (Ungerleider & Mishkin, 1982), and neuropsychological techniques (Gross, Rocha-Miranda, & Bender, 1972; Mountcastle, Lynch, & Georgopoulos, 1975; Rolls et al, 1982, Rolls, Baylis, & Leonards, 1985, Hubel & Livingstone, 1987).

Memory

Progress in the field of memory has been no less significant. First, there is the finding that multiple neural structures from numerous brain regions and hierarchies (for example, association cortices of different orders, cortical limbic system structures, basal forebrain nuclei, thalamic nuclei) must act together in a concerted action for learning and retrieval to occur (see, Corkin, 1984; A. Damasio et al, 1985a and b; Squire et al. 1987). Second, there is the demonstration

---

FIGURE 2.9. CT of a 74-year-old, right-handed man who suddenly developed what was described as "blurry vision." A formal visual field defect could not be detected, but objects "appeared and disappeared" erratically from either visual field. This made it difficult for him to read or to look at objects and faces the examiners pointed to. It was obvious, however, that whenever an image fell into sharp "focus," it was seen readily and could be recognized, identified, and named (this occurred for objects, faces, and words). For instance, his description of the "Cookie Theft" picture (from the Boston Diagnostic Aphasia Examination) was labored because he could only give accurate and detailed descriptions of fragments of the picture, appreciated in unsystematic order. After a few seconds, he would report that the particular fragment had "disappeared" and that something else was now in its place. This is typical of the defects known as visual disorientation, as first described by Gordon Holmes (1918b). Its consequence is the phenomenon of simultanagnosia, the inability to appreciate more than one aspect of the visual panorama at any single time. The individual cannot experience a spatially coherent visual field.

A CT obtained with injection of contrast material (A) shows bilateral areas of increased density corresponding to the damaged areas. These are seen mainly in the higher cuts, mostly corresponding to the supracalcarine association cortices. The post-mortem images (B) obtained two weeks after the CT confirmed the presence of small cortical infarcts in the supracalcarine watershed region of both hemispheres.

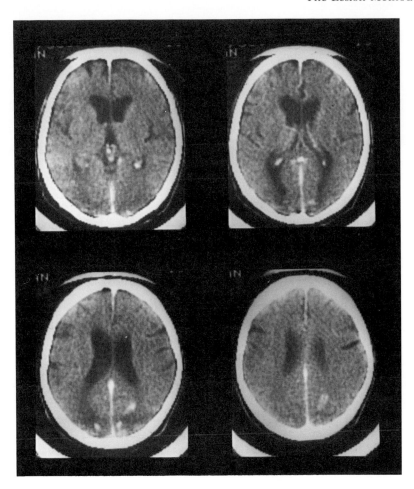

(A)

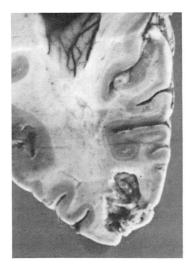
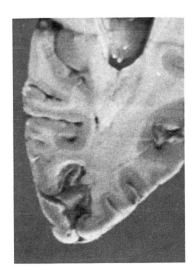

(B)

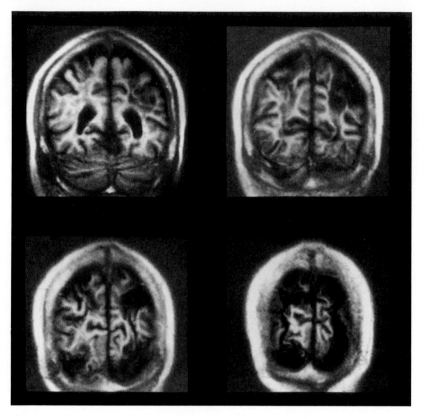

(A)

FIGURE 2.10. MR of a 54-year-old, right-handed man who suddenly developed visual disorientation just as described in Figure 2.9. In addition, however, he also developed a difficulty in hand-reaching of objects under visual guidance. The aiming of the hand toward a target was no longer accurate. There was a striking difference between the way the patient could correctly bring his index finger to the tip of his nose (with either the right or the left hand) and his inability to reach a visual target with precision. Reaching the nose required no visual guidance and was normal. Reaching a visual target placed in a novel location did require visual update and was impaired. He would generally fall short of the target, attempting to correct the approach by small tentative movements reminiscent of those a blind person would perform in similar circumstances. This deficit is known as optic ataxia. The combination of optic ataxia and visual disorientation, together with yet another sign, ocular apraxia, constitutes the Balint syndrome (Balint, 1909). (Ocular apraxia is the inability to shift

that *domains of knowledge* (for example, knowledge for different types of objects, faces, language, social behavior), and *levels of knowledge complexity* (for example, ranging from unique and subordinate, to generic and supraordinate) are important factors according to which memory's neural substrates must be organized (A. Damasio, 1989 a and b; A. Damasio, H. Damasio, & Tranel, 1989; Warrington & Shallice, 1984). Third, there is the mounting evidence that the neural substrates on which representations of external stimuli are perceived and can be reevoked must be different from those structures that contain the binding codes on the basis of which representations

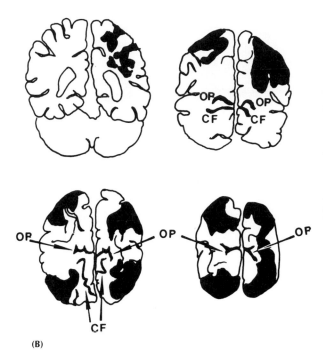

(B)

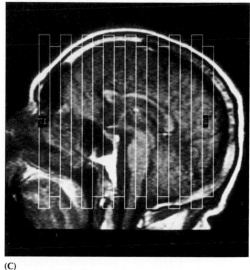

(C)

one's gaze towards a new stimulus willfully.) Neither this patient nor the previous one showed any difficulty in color perception, or visual recognition of words, objects, and faces.

The lesions are bilateral and fall both in the supracalcarine association cortices and posterior parietal regions. (A and B) Note that these coronal cuts were obtained with the head hyperextended (see the pilot scan in C). This means that cut number 4 (last cut) shows the occipitoparietal sulcus (OP) dividing the brain regions into parietal lobe, above, and supracalcarine occipital lobe, below. The calcarine fissure itself (CF) can be seen in cuts number 2 and 3 only. The areas of damage are above and at the level of CF, but not below. Investigators in our group are now studying these patients with experimental attention paradigms in order to explore the components of attentional mechanisms that are disrupted by differently placed occipito-parietal lesions.

can be reconstructed and reexperienced (A. Damasio, 1989 a and b; A. Damasio et al, 1985a; A. Damasio, H. Damasio, & Tranel, 1989).

The study of the agnosias—which in reality are nothing but restricted amnesias caused by a defect in single modality triggering of memory—has revealed intriguing dissociations among the categories for which learning and recognition are precluded. For instance, a result of damage circumscribed to certain sectors of the visual association cortices, subjects may lose their ability to recognize visually the identity of human faces (they can recognize the voices behind

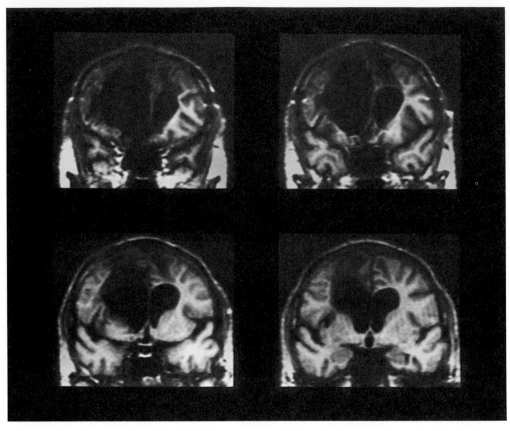

(A)

FIGURE 2.11. T$_1$ weighted MR (A) and correspond-ing templates (B) of a 48-year-old man. To remove a large frontal meningioma, four years earlier, a significant surgical resection of frontal cortices was necessary. After surgery, there were marked changes in the patient's personality. These have remained to this day and affect his social conduct, decision-making, and planning.

In brief, he fails to recognize the significance of otherwise obvious clues in social situations. He thus makes highly unwise decisions in matters re-garding friendships, financial transactions, profes-sional conduct, and so on. He also fails to recog-nize that he does have problems in these areas (anosognosia). His intellectual abilities, as mea-sured by neuropsychological tests, were and still are superior. His memory is normal for domains of knowledge not related to social information and

those faces) but they will not lose the ability to recognize the mean-ing of facial expressions, or to recognize faces as faces (Tranel, A. Damasio, & H. Damasio, 1988.) In other words, recognition of unique identity but not of category is precluded. Although the defect in unique recognition applies to virtually every other entity—build-ings, vehicles, personal effect, etc.—the preservation of category recognition is violated in certain instances. For example, the ability to recognize carpentry tools visually may be preserved, whereas that of recognizing musical instruments may be precluded, notwith-standing the fact that both musical instruments and carpentry tools

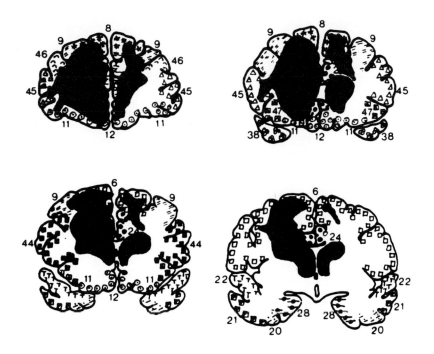

(B)

conduct (his current Memory Quotient is 142). His language is also entirely normal. His Wisconsin card-sorting test performance is excellent. (For other details, see Eslinger & Damasio, 1985.) He is perhaps the most striking case of this sort of knowledge domain dissociation on record.

The MR shows the extent of damage in his frontal cortices. The lesion is more extensive on the right, where the mesial frontal lobe and its white matter are largely destroyed. The lateral cortices are spared. The region of basal forebrain is spared (see lower left cut). On the left, the damage is more restricted, involving part of the mesial surface and only the immediately underlying white matter. Again, the lateral cortices and the basal forebrain region are spared. Patients such as this are currently part of a study on the neural basis of "acquired sociopathy."

are man-made and manipulable objects. (A. Damasio, H. Damasio, & Tranel, 1989). Furthermore, these same agnosic patients may recognize the unique identity of the persons whose faces have become meaningless, by watching their characteristic gait or postures, an ability that testifies to the possibility of gaining access to identifying memoranda that are clearly stored separately from the stimulus for which recognition is requested. (A. Damasio, H. Damasio, & Tranel 1988). Such findings demonstrate that the organization of knowledge honors different categories of reality as based on different physical structures and different interactions between perceiver and

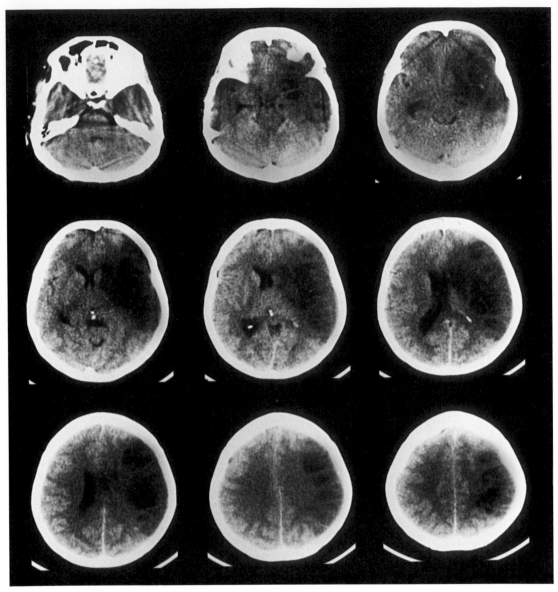

(A)

FIGURE 2.12. CT (A) and corresponding templates (B) of a 34-year-old woman, obtained a few hours after she developed left hemiplegia and severe left visuospatial neglect. She appeared unaware of her defects, specifically denying that there was any-thing wrong with her left limb (anosognosia). Note that most of the territory of the right middle cerebral artery is occupied by an area of decreased density. This includes cortex and white matter in the frontal, temporal, and parietal lobes, as well

external structure. These findings also point to the importance of the channel used to reach memory banks, and provide evidence for the separation of memory by level of complexity. There is a preservation of the access to knowledge on the basis of which an entity can be categorized at the *basic object level* (a face as a face), or at the

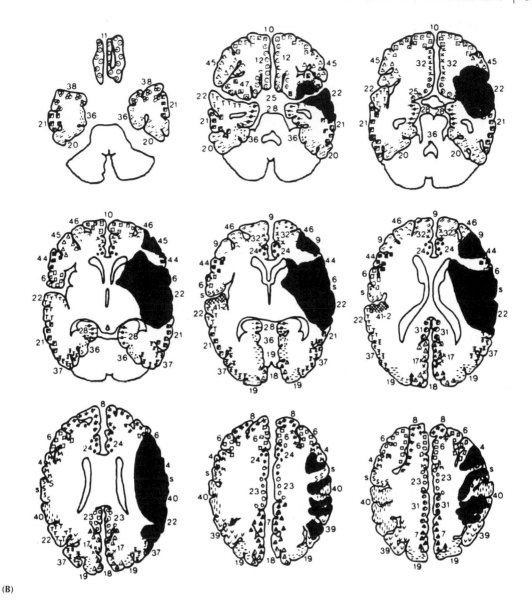

(B)

as the insula and the region of the basal ganglia. The lesion spares the thalamus. The margins of this low-density area are ill-defined, as is often the case with recent infarcts. The ventricular system is deviated to the left, a typical sign of edema. At this stage, it is not possible to discriminate the infarcted areas from the areas of edema (see also Figure 3.28 and 3.29 for a later scan of the same patient).

supraordinate level (a face as evidence of membership in the human species, or in the animal world, or in the kingdom of living things). Such categorical knowledge is usually referred to as *generic* or *categorical memory* (our terms), or *semantic memory* (the term introduced by Tulving in 1972). On the other hand, the specific knowledge

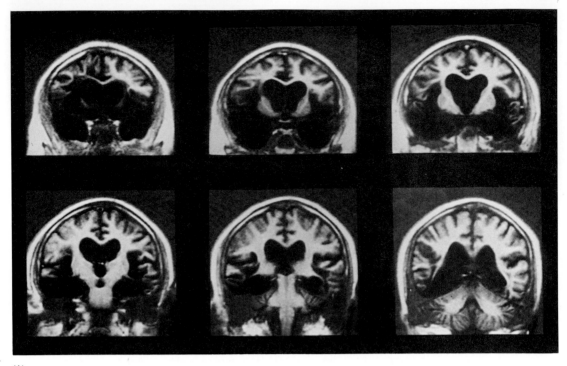

(A)

FIGURE 2.13. T$_1$ weighted MR (A) and corresponding templates (B) of a 57-year-old man who had
herpes simplex encephalitis 10 years earlier. At the
time of this MR, the patient had a profound global
amnesia and a pervasive defect of olfaction. The
amnesia was complete for episodic material, but
left intact most generic material and perceptuo-
motor skills. It covered both the anterograde and
the retrograde components of memory; that is, he
could not recall or recognize *any* episodic information from his entire past nor could he recall or
recognize information that might have been
learned since the time of lesion onset.

Note the complete destruction of the anterior
temporal regions (including the amygdala, hippocampus, parahippocampal gyrus, the region of the
temporal pole (area 38), and the anterior portion
of the inferior, middle, and superior temporal gyri

necessary to characterize a stimulus at *subordinate level* (for example,
the unique face of a friend) is not accessible, that is, the specific
memories needed for unique identifications are not evocable. Such
specific and unique knowledge is usually referred to as *episodic memory*, a term also introduced by Tulving. (The terms *supraordinate*,
basic object, and *subordinate*, which qualify taxonomic levels, come from
Rosch's work on categorization: Rosch et al, 1976). The difference
between memories recalled at generic level or episodic level is one
of complexity and is related to the quantity of evoked items necessary for the establishment of the temporal or spatial markings on
the basis of which unique identities are defined.

Other striking examples of domain specificity in memory occur
with some lesions of the frontal cortices, which can preclude the
automatic access of memories related to knowledge of social behav-

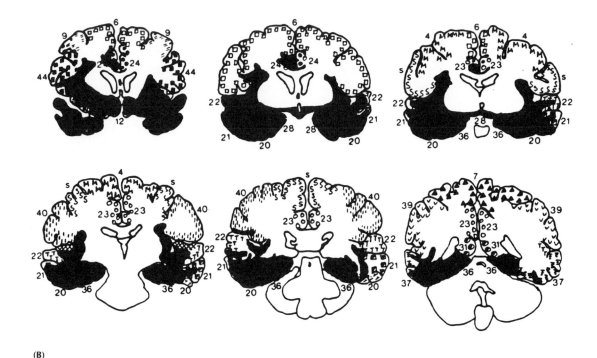

(B)

(areas 20, 21, and anterior 22). From the level of the primary auditory cortices, onward, the superior temporal gyrus is spared bilaterally. The left middle temporal gyrus is also mostly preserved.

Note that the basal ganglia and the thalamus are entirely preserved, as are all of the occipital and parietal cortices and most of the frontal cortices (with the exception of the most caudal orbital region).

The basal forebrain region and the insula are also damaged bilaterally. Patients with this pattern of damage (or with damage in sectors of this region) are prime subjects for cognitive experiments probing mechanisms of learning, recall, and recognition.

iors (A. Damasio & Tranel, 1988; Tranel, A. Damasio, & H. Damasio, 1988), while preserving the access to all other domains and levels of complexity of knowledge; or with lesions to right parietal cortices, which impair access to memory of body states. Striking examples of the latter can be found in so-called anosognosia (Anderson & Tranel, 1988) [see Figure 2.11, 2.12 and also 3.28 and 3.29]. Naturally, the most dramatic example of domain-specific memory organization is verbal knowledge, especially knowledge of the lexicon and grammar. Its disruption causes some of the well-known aphasias.

Patients with damage in anterior temporal structures involving the hippocampus, the overlying entorhinal cortex, and the region of the amygdala, develop major learning defects and defects of retrieval of previously formed memories. Just as in the case of agnosics, these patients' difficulties with recognition and recall mostly involve the domain of complex episodic knowledge necessary for unique identification of entities or events, while sparing the ability to recognize or recall the broader categories to which entities or events belong. On the other hand, unlike agnosics, these patients' defects pertain to all sensory modalities and no channel of access is spared selectively (A. Damasio et al, 1985a Milner, Corkin, & Teuber, 1968) [see Figure 2.13]. A knowledge domain spared in such patients is that of perceptuo-motor skills, such as mirror tracing and rotor pursuit, which require a motor response rather than the experience of internally evoked factual knowledge (Cohen & Squire, 1980; Eslinger & Damasio, 1986; Milner, Corkin, & Teuber, 1968).

The acquisition and retrieval of memory requires the participation of multiple neural structures of different hierarchies. This has been brought to light by the description of memory impairments following not only damage to the mesial temporal cortices, but also to (a) the basal forebrain region that contains the septal nuclei, the diagonal brand of Broca, and the substantia innominata, within which a large part of the nucleus basalis of Meynert is located (see A. Damasio et al, 1985b; Alexander & Freeman, 1983); (b) the nonmesial anterotemporal cortices (within areas 38, 20, 21, 22, and part of 37) and the insular cortices; (c) the thalamus, especially in its dorsomedial sector, involving not only the dorsomedial nuclei but also the nonspecific nuclei close to the midline, such as the nucleus reuniens and the centrum medianum (Kritchevsky, Graff-Radford, & A. Damasio 1987; Mair, Warrington, & Weiskrantz, 1979; Squire et al, 1987; Victor, Adams & Collins, 1988); and (d) the hypothalamus (Victor, Adams, & Collins, 1988).

Language

The study of language disorders using the lesion method has been especially rewarding. Until a decade ago, the neurology of language remained confined to the perisylvian area, but new studies based on the lesion method have taken it beyond that region and even revised traditional concepts pertaining to that sector of the brain.

Prominent among the developments is the role now accorded to subcortical gray matter in language processes. The classical aphasia types were linked to lesions in the cerebral cortex or the directly subjacent white matter. Now there is evidence that aphasia can follow damage to deep gray matter structures of the left hemisphere. These structures include the basal ganglia, a set of central gray nuclei that until recently had been considered to be a purely motor structure (Aran et al, 1983; A. Damasio et al, 1982a; Brunner et al, 1982; H. Damasio, Eslinger, & Adams 1984; Naeser et al, 1982), and the anterolateral nuclei of the thalamus (Graff-Radford et al,

1984, 1985) [see Figures 2.14 and 2.15]. The findings have established the region of the head of the caudate in the left hemisphere as a critical component in the anatomical network that sustains language (damage to the left putamen, another major sector of the basal ganglia located nearby, does not cause aphasia, a clear indication of the specificity of the lesion). Given the neuroanatomical and neurophysiological characterization of this region in nonhuman primates, it appears that damage to the caudate indirectly disrupts cortical processes involved in perceptual organization (especially in relation to auditory stimuli) and motor programming (A. Damasio, 1983, 1985c).

Another development concerns the role of the limbic system and of higher-order association cortices in language. The limbic system is an aggregate of cortical structures (located in the internal surface of the temporal and frontal cortices) and of subcortical nuclei placed near the forebrain's midline. Although the system plays a crucial role in memory, attention, and the regulation of emotion and affect, it had not been implicated in language until Geschwind hypothesized that a connection between the multimodal cortices in the left angular gyrus and the left mesial temporal region would be crucial for learning vocabulary (Geschwind, 1965). Now, evidence exists that his hypothesis was correct. Damage to the left anterior temporal lobe (which contain the hippocampus as well as its afferent and efferent staging areas) is associated with severe verbal learning defects (Corkin, 1984; A. Damasio et al, 1985a; Hyman et al, 1984; Milner, 1966; Van Hoesen & Damasio, 1987). In addition to a role in the learning of new lexicon, evidence exists that the left hippocampus, along with interconnected higher-order multimodal cortices (in areas 37, 20, 21, and 38), is also involved in retrieval of selected lexical categories but not in phonemic or syntactical levels of language operation (H. Damasio, 1988; Tranel, A. Damasio, & H. Damasio, 1988; Van Hoesen & A. Damasio, 1987).

Few issues illustrate progress in aphasiology better than the recent history of studies in conduction aphasia. Its status as a distinct aphasia type was established in the 1960s (Benton et al, 1973; Goodglass & Kaplan, 1972; Kertesz, 1979). However, its anatomical correlates and the classical account of its cardinal clinical sign, the impairment of repetition, have undergone significant revisions. The condition is now attributed to one of two dominant anatomical loci: (a) damage to area 40 (supramarginal gyrus) with or without extension to subinsular white matter [see Figure 2.16]; (b) damage to primary auditory cortices (areas 41 and 42) with extension into the insular cortex and underlying white matter, but sparing of all or most of area 22 posteriorly (H. Damasio, 1988; H. Damasio & A. Damasio, 1980; Rubens & Selnes, 1986). No evidence supports Wernicke's original hypothesis that this aphasia would be caused by a

FIGURE 2.14. Chronic CT (A) of a 54-year-old, right-handed man who suddenly developed a right hemiparesis and aphasia eight months earlier. At the time the CT was obtained, the patient had nonfluent speech with a mild dysarthria. He made frequent semantic and phonemic paraphasias. Yet he would often produce fairly long and grammatically organized sentences (five to 10 words). Aural comprehension of sentences was severely defective and sentence repetition was compromised. This aphasia profile did not fit any of the established aphasia categories. The combination of long word strings ("fluent" sentences) with dysarthria is uncommon. The combination of right hemiparesis and severe auditory comprehension disturbance is also unusual. The profile is certainly "atypical."

The CT image is that of a stable stroke in the territory of the left lenticulo-striate arteries (the small penetrating arteries that take off from the stem of the middle cerebral artery). It damages the head of the left caudate nucleus, the anterior limb of the internal capsule, and the putamen. Both the frontal horn of the lateral ventricle and the sylvian fissure are markedly dilated. This is the result of retraction of brain tissue caused by resolution of the infarction.

Dilatation ex-vacuum is a fairly constant and relatively early phenomenon following infarcts in this region (see H. Damasio et al, 1984). Note the absence of damage in the language-related cortices of the left frontal and left temporo-parietal regions.

This image is quite representative of aphasia-causing infarctions in the left basal ganglia. Mirror image infarctions in the right basal ganglia region cause left hemiparesis, left neglect, but no aphasia.

Chronic MR (B and C) (T$_1$ weighted images) of a 67-year-old, right-handed woman who suddenly developed a right hemiparesis and some speech articulation difficulties three months earlier. At the time this MR scan was obtained, her speech was well-articulated, fluent, and free of phonemic or semantic paraphasias. Aural comprehension of sentences, reading comprehension, and sentence repetition were entirely normal.

Both coronal and transverse MR cuts show a small infarction in the posterior limb of the internal capsule. The infarction extends into the very posterior and superior region of the putamen, which is otherwise spared. There is no sign of damage in either the head of the caudate nucleus or the anterior limb of the capsule.

Left basal ganglia lesions that spare the head of the caudate do not

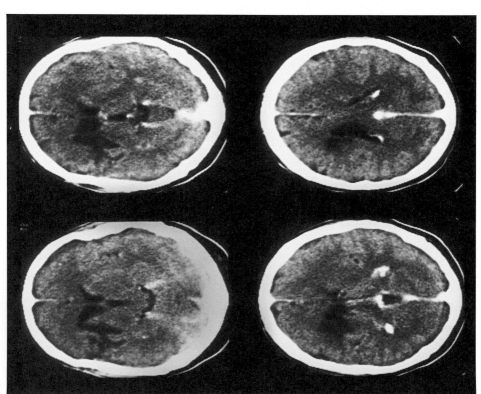

(A)

40

cause linguistic defects. Lesions involving the left putamen may or may not cause dysarthria and dysprosody.

The core neuroanatomical and neuropsychological characterization of aphasic patients is critical to the interpretation of experiments in which cognitive and linguistic variables are manipulated.

(C)

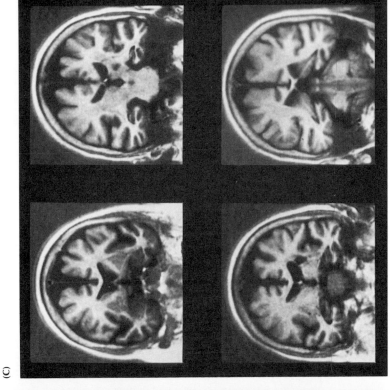

(B)

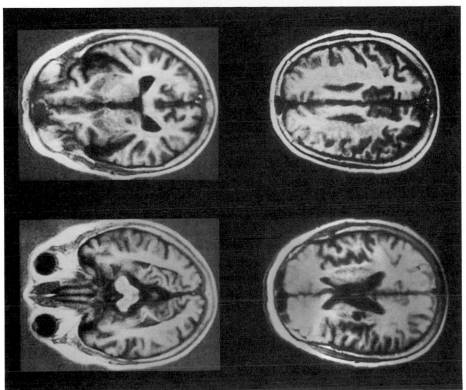

41

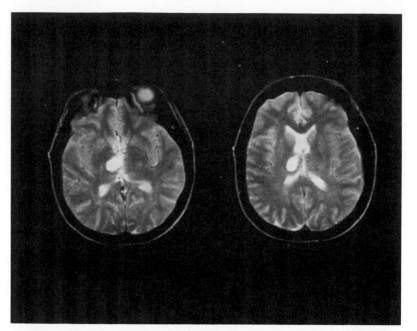

(A)

(B)

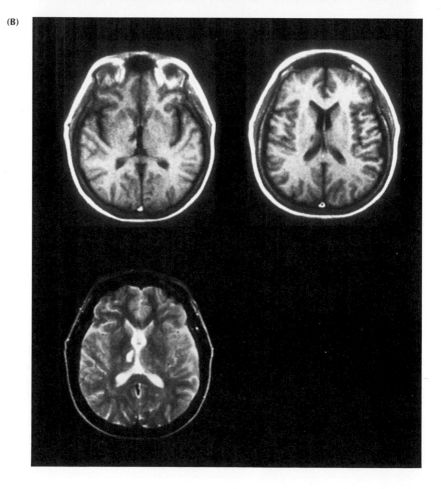

lesion of *only* the white matter connecting Wernicke's area to Broca's. Damage virtually always involves a critical cortical sector and is thus a "center aphasia," in Wernicke's terminology, just as much as Broca's aphasia or Wernicke's aphasia are. The damage does consistently involve some white matter connections, as is true in any aphasia, and those connections are part of a large sheath of complex circuitry that conjoin temporal, parietal, and frontal cortices (Galaburda & Pandya, 1983); that projection system contains, in its dorsal sector, the classical arcuate fasciculus that was originally linked to conduction aphasia. Wernicke's notion, later revived by Konorski and Geschwind (Konorski, Kozniewska & Stepien 1961, Geschwind 1965), that the repetition defect would be caused by the interruption of that tract alone is not tenable. Even less credible is the classical pathophysiological account of the problem: the "blocking" of an echoic, one-step communication device from an acoustic to a motor processor. The repetition defect is more fittingly explained by the disruption of a multistep and *not* unidirectional process that, while leading from auditory perception to motor implementation, requires the perception of phoneme clusters, their holding in short-term memory, and their activation and assembly in articulatory phonetic patterns.

The lesion method has contributed significantly to the understanding of global aphasia, a major clinical presentation of language disorder. The traditional correlates of global aphasia comprise (a) the anterior language region, as in Broca's aphasia; (b) the entire basal ganglia complex; (c) the insula and auditory cortices, as in conduction aphasia; and (d) the posterior language-related cortices (posterior area 22, lateral area 37, areas 40 and 39), as in Wernicke's aphasia (H. Damasio, 1981, 1988; Kertesz, 1979; Naeser & Hayward, 1978). Global aphasics with a continuous single locus of damage encompassing all of those areas are severely aphasic from the outset and show little or no improvement [Figure 2.17]. Recently,

---

FIGURE 2.15. MR of a 47-year-old, right-handed woman who suddenly became confused and aphasic. The confusion rapidly cleared and 10 days after onset she was alert and oriented to person. Spontaneously, she spoke softly and made minimal paraphasic errors. However, laboratory studies revealed a severe word-finding difficulty and disclosed numerous semantic paraphasias. Reading aloud also led to paraphasias. Her visual naming ability, auditory comprehension of sentences, and ability to generate word lists from an initial letter were all severely defective. On the other hand, sentence repetition, reading for comprehension, and writing were only moderately impaired. Her nonverbal abilities were normal. Three months later, she was remarkably better in all aspects of language.

This clinical picture is often encountered in patients with left thalamic damage with the location described below. After confusion clears, an aphasia with intact repetition becomes the dominant disturbance.

Both the acute T_2 weighted MR (A) and the chronic T_1 and T_2 weighted MR (B) show an area of infarct in the anterior region of the left thalamus.

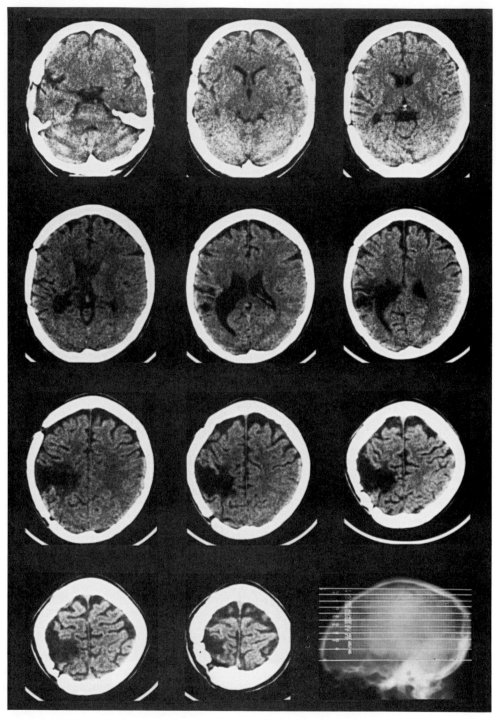

(A)

FIGURE 2.16. Chronic CT (A) and corresponding templates (B) of a patient who, seven years before this study, underwent resection of an arteriovenous malformation in the left parietal region. The low-density area localized to the left supramar-ginal gyrus is the result of the resection. The patient showed the typical defects associated with conduction aphasia. Acutely, she had fluent speech with phonemic paraphasias and occasional semantic paraphasias. On occasion, she had word-

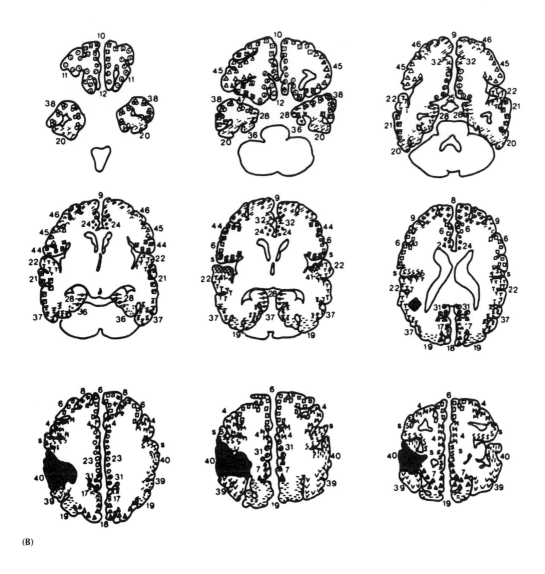

(B)

finding difficulty and would produce successive approximations to her intended verbal target ("conduites d'approche"). The production of specific names, as is required in Benton's Visual Naming Test, was particularly apt to bring out this deficit. Comprehension of colloquial speech was intact and she carried out verbal commands normally, even if laboratory assessment of complex sentence comprehension was defective. Digit and sentence repetition were grossly defective. At the time this CT was obtained, she had recovered remarkably but still had occasional difficulty in producing specific names and still used "conduite d'approche." Her repetition remained defective.

She continues to show a complete left ear extinction in dichotic listening.

The defect is entirely confined to the anterior portion of the inferior parietal lobule (the supramarginal gyrus or Brodmann's area 40). Note that spared areas include both the primary auditory cortices within Heschl's gyri, which can be seen on the fourth cut (first cut on second row), and the posterior portion of the superior temporal gyrus (area 22 or Wernicke's area), seen immediately behind Heschl's gyri and in the following cut (A). (See also Figure 4.7 for another example of conduction aphasia).

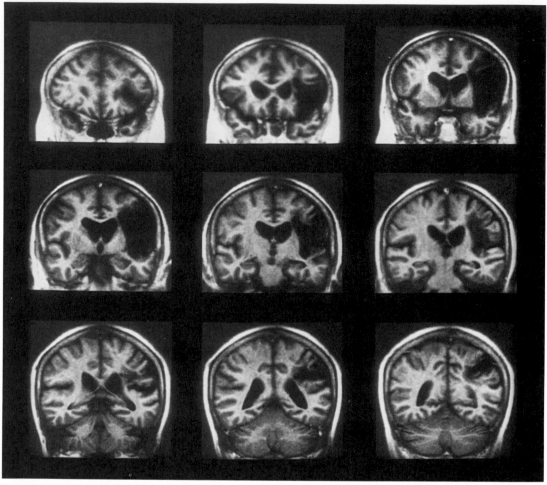

(A)

FIGURE 2.17(I). T$_1$ weighted MR (A) and corresponding templates (B) of a 60-year-old, right-handed man who had sudden onset of right hemiparesis and severe aphasia one year earlier. The motor deficit involved mainly the right upper extremity and face. Language output was limited to a stereotype. He was unable to repeat even single words, including his name, and showed a marked defect in the auditory comprehension of sentences. He was unable to read or write (agraphia was severe, even with the left hand). Attempts at singing improved his ability to use language only minimally. At the time this MR was obtained, his oral communication was still marred by severely dysarthric and paraphasic nonfluent speech. Auditory comprehension was defective, even for simple items of colloquial conversation. He remained severely impaired in virtually all aspects of linguistic performance. However, nonlinguistic abilities were in the low/normal range. This is the classical clinical picture of global aphasia, a condition that is now known to be caused by different patterns of left hemisphere damage. One of those patterns is described below.

The MR shows a large, well-defined area of low signal in the left hemisphere occupying a large

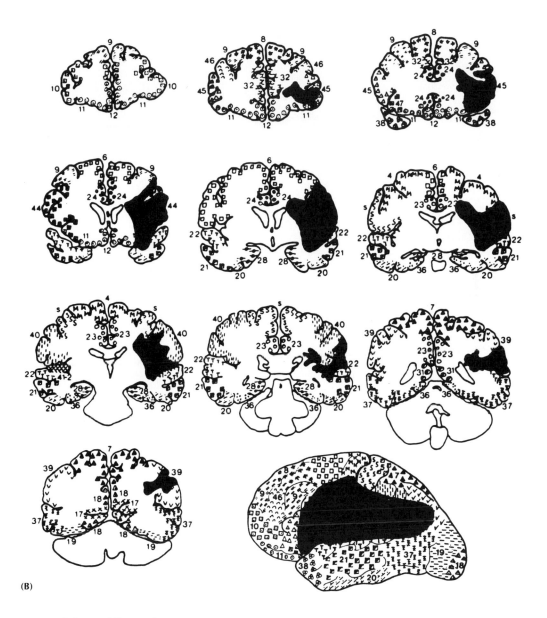

(B)

sector of the middle cerebral artery territory. This includes cortical and subcortical white matter in (a) most of the frontal operculum (areas 44 and 45 or Broca's area), (b) the lower portion of the rolandic cortices, (c) most of the inferior parietal lobule (area 40, or Supramarginal gyrus, and area 39, or angular gyrus), (d) most of the superior temporal gyrus, including the transverse gyri of Heschl, and (e) the insula and possibly most lateral portion of the lenticular nucleus.

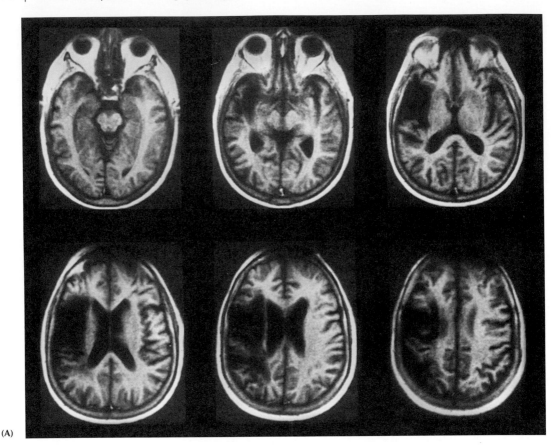

(A)

FIGURE 2.17(II). Transverse cuts of the T₁ weighted MR shown in Figure 2.17(I). MR transparencies shown in (A) and corresponding templates in (B).

however, other patients have been described whose inaugural presentation is that of a global aphasia but who do *not* have hemiplegia and who improve dramatically. Such patients have *two* noncontiguous foci of damage, one in the frontal lobe and another in the temporo-parietal region, sparing a wide area of motor- and language-related structures (H. Damasio, 1981, 1988; Tranel et al, 1987; Vignolo, Boccardi, & Caverni, 1986) [See Figure 2.18]. Still another group of patients initially presenting with global aphasia and contralateral motor deficits may show recovery, but to a limited extent. These are patients who present with large frontal lobe lesions with extension into basal ganglia on parietal lobe, but spare all temporal structures. Such patients often evolve rather rapidly into Broca's aphasia [see Figure 2.19]. Figures 2.20 and 2.21 illustrate the more typical image of Broca's aphasia.

The lesion method has also permitted the study of the aphasia for American Sign Language (ASL) and the discovery that such aphasias are caused by dysfunction to the left hemisphere (Bellugi,

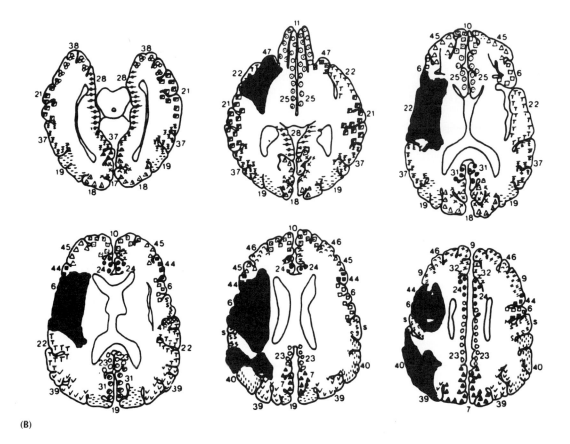

(B)

Poizner, & Klima, 1983; A. Damasio et al, 1986; Poizner, Bellugi, & Klima, 1987), suggesting that the nonauditory-based languages are as linked to the left hemisphere as auditory-based ones. The ASL aphasias are structurally comparable to the major aphasias encountered in non-sign languages, and their types correlate with lesion location in the traditional fashion.

Finally, a series of lesion studies have also established that the cortices in the hemispheres' mesial surfaces, although crucial for the initiation and maintenance of movement (including the movement used in speech) (Alexander & Schmitt, 1980; A. Damasio & Van Hoesen, 1980, 1983; H. Damasio, 1981, 1988; Freedman, Alexander, & Naeser, 1984; Laplane, Talairach, & Meininger, 1977; Ross, Damasio, & Eslinger, 1986), do not cause true aphasia. These cortices influence many aspects of cognition and behavior beyond language. Rather, damage in these areas causes true mutism and akinesia. Patients fail to communicate by word and by gesture, and experience a virtual state of avolition [see Figure 2.22].

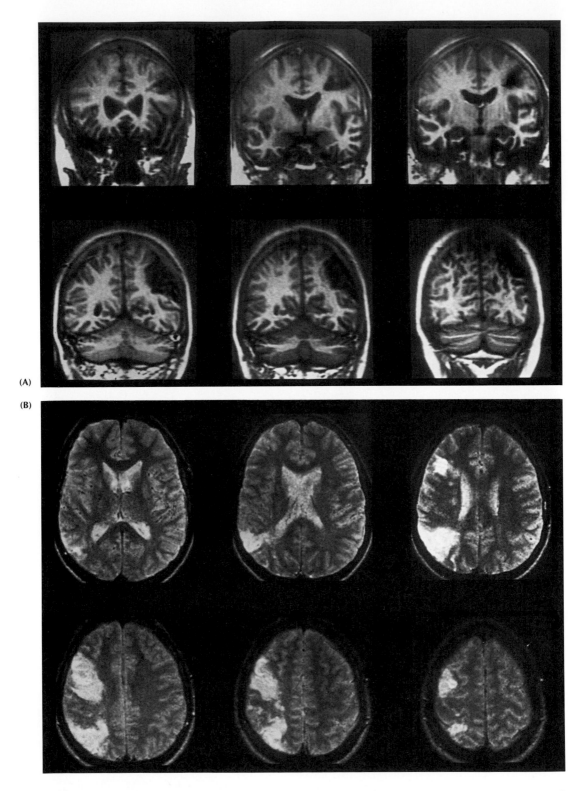

(A)

(B)

FIGURE 2.18. Chronic MR (A and B) and corresponding templates (C) of a 37-year-old, right-handed man who suddenly became unable to speak while playing a game of golf. He developed *no motor deficit* and, in fact, was able to complete the game. Yet he was severely aphasic and his

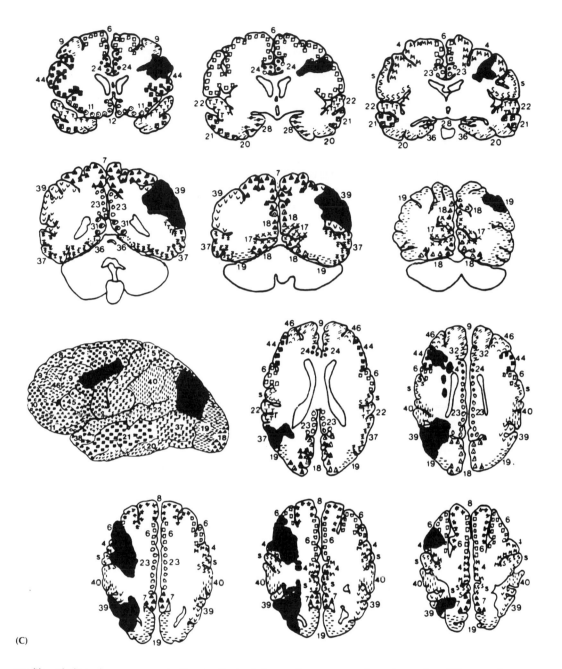

(C)

profile of disturbance was similar to that of the patient in Figure 2.17. In the first week, he had no spontaneous speech and he attempted to respond to questions by producing grunts and gestures. Formal testing revealed severely defective performance in virtually all language aspects, but intact nonverbal abilities. At the time this MR was obtained, however, five months post-onset, he was able to produce long and grammatically correct sentences without paraphasic errors.

Considering that the early profile is that of global aphasia and the prognosis of global aphasia is poor,

the recovery is noteworthy. When such recovery takes place, the atomical basis of the global aphasia is likely to be atypical, as was the case in this patient.

The MR (coronal T_1 weighted images in [A] and transverse T_2 weighted images in [B]) shows that there are two independent areas of infarct, one in the frontal lobe and another in the parietal lobe. In other words, there are two discontinuous foci of damage, rather than one continuous lesion. The frontal lesion damages the superior portion of the frontal operculum (area 44) and extends superiorly and posteriorly into the pre-motor cortex. The posterior lesion damages mainly the angular gyrus (area 39). Most of the language-related cortices, both in the frontal operculum (areas 45 and part of 44) and in the temporo-parietal region (areas 41 and 42, posterior area 22, and supramarginal gyrus or area 40) are spared. The intactness of these areas

explains the dramatic improvement of linguistic abilities in this and in other patients. The sparing of rolandic cortices (motor area 4 and somatosensory areas 3, 1, and 2), and of the basal ganglia and internal capsule, explains the lack of motor signs.

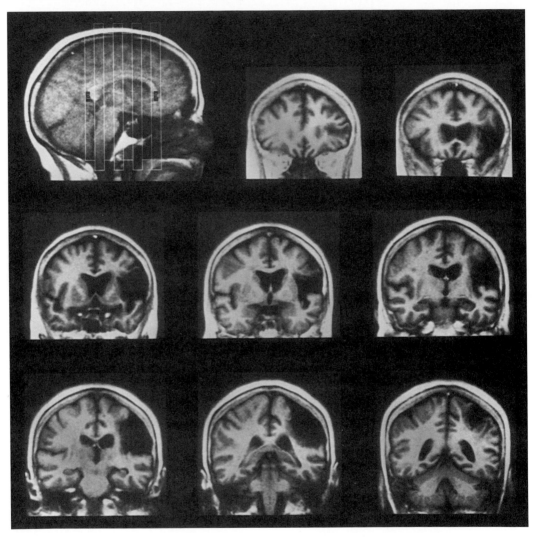

(A)

FIGURE 2.19(I). T$_1$ weighted MR (A) and corresponding templates (B) of a 67-year-old, left-handed woman (Oldfield-Geschwind questionnaire score of −50) who had developed right hemiparesis and mutism two years earlier. Within three weeks of onset, her complete mutism had given way to effortful and sparse speech, mainly consisting of stereotypes. She was severely impaired in virtually all linguistic tasks. At the time, her neuropsychological profile was that of a global aphasia. By the

time this MR was obtained, her speech was nonfluent, effortful, with severe word-finding difficulty, and paraphasic (both semantic and phonemic paraphasias). Her sentence repetition was defective. Prosody and articulation were only mildly impaired and she often could communicate by writing, although she made spelling mistakes. Comprehension of simple sentences had improved markedly, but comprehension of grammatically elaborate sentences was still severely de-

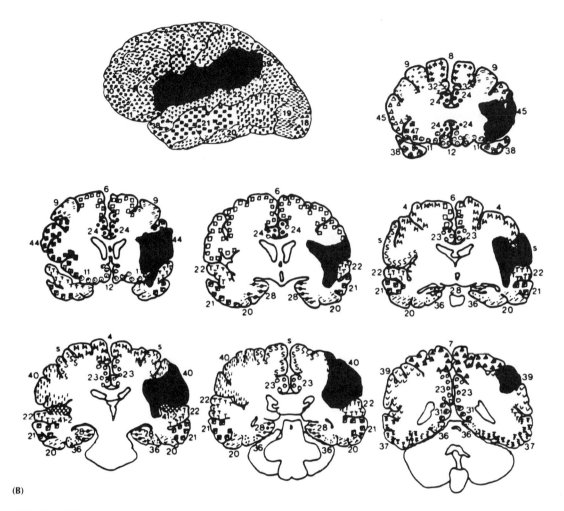

(B)

FIGURE 2.19(I) *continued.*

fective. By then, the neuropsychological profile largely conformed to the category of Broca's aphasia. The anatomical pattern is one of several variants that can be noted in association with these symptoms. Note that although Wernicke's area is spared, the lesion does trespass well beyond the frontal region usually compromised in Broca's aphasia. This pattern explains the initial global aphasia picture and its subsequent evolution.

MR shows a large, well-defined area of low sig-

nal that involves the cortex and subcortical white matter in the frontal and parietal lobes. As in the previous case, the lesion involves the frontal operculum, but here, not all of Broca's area is destroyed. The lower portion of the rolandic cortices, the anterior supramarginal gyrus, and the insula are damaged, but the basal ganglia are spared. The angular gyrus and all of the temporal lobe are intact, including Wernicke's area.

Figures 4.21 and 4.22 show the acute MR of a similar patient.

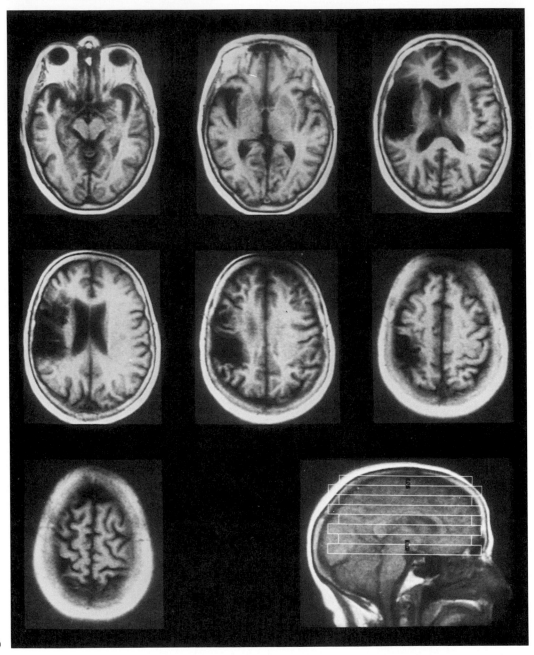

(A)

FIGURE 2.19(II). Transverse cuts of the MR seen in Figure 2.19(I). T_1 weighted transparencies are shown in A and the corresponding templates in B. Note that the intactness of the temporal lobe is more readily recognized in coronal (2.19[I]) than transverse cuts.

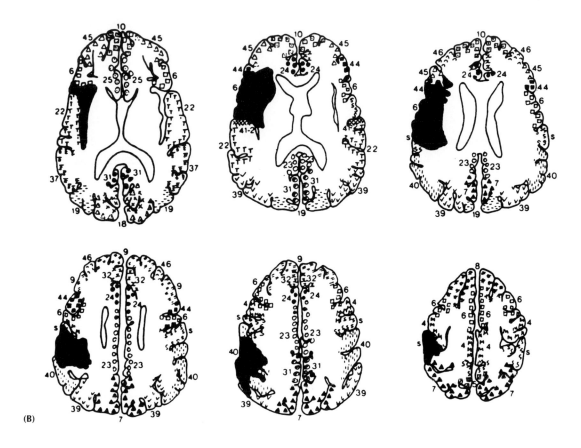

(B)

Multiregional Time-Locked Retroactivation: A Model for Neural Systems Subtending Cognition

Framework and Overall Design

The main source for the concepts in this model was our personal study of cognitive changes in several hundred patients with focal brain lesions. Agnosic, amnesic, aphasic, and so-called "frontal lobe" patients constituted the majority of the sample. The thrust for the model came from the realization that available accounts of the neural basis of cognition, for instance, those implicit in center localization-ism, behaviorism, functional equipotentiality, or disconnection syndrome theory, are no longer satisfactory to interpret the consequences of focal brain damage on cognition.

The focus of the model is the nature of the experiences that constitute perception or are conjured up in recall and recognition. The model discusses a possible structure and organization behind the cerebral inscription of such experiences, at the anatomic-physiological level of systems.

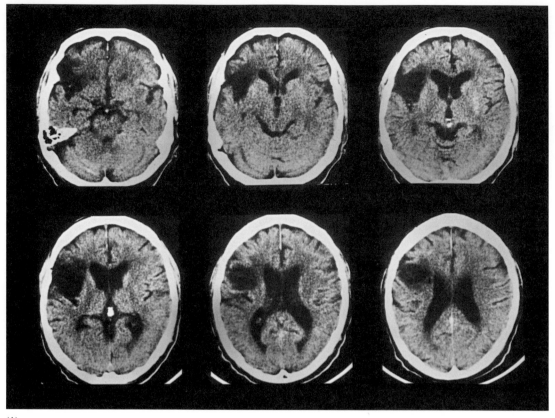

(A)

FIGURE 2.20. CT (A) and corresponding templates (B) of a 76-year-old, right-handed man who, three months earlier, developed marked aphasia accompanied by a mild and transient hemiparesis. His speech was severely nonfluent (spontaneous speech was limited to three-word sentences) and had profuse semantic paraphasias. Articulation was defective. He gestured frequently and appropriately when attempting to speak. He was able to sing. He was able to follow simple verbal commands. At the time of this CT, speech remained nonfluent, paraphasic, and poorly articulated. He was unable to repeat sentences. His performance on formal language tasks had improved but was still defective, most notably in the use of grammatical knowledge to arrive at the meaning of sentences. In traditional terms, this presentation conforms to the clinical category of Broca's aphasia. Recovery was poor.

The CT shows a well-defined area of low density in the left frontal lobe, involving a large portion of the frontal operculum and underlying white matter. The lesion extends to surrounding premotor areas and to most of the insula.

Note that our use of diagnostic categories such as "Broca aphasia" does not signify acceptance of the physiopathologic mechanisms traditionally invoked to explain language defects. The syndrome labels are crutches for communication, the same way that core neuroanatomy and neuropsychology are a base for additional experiments.

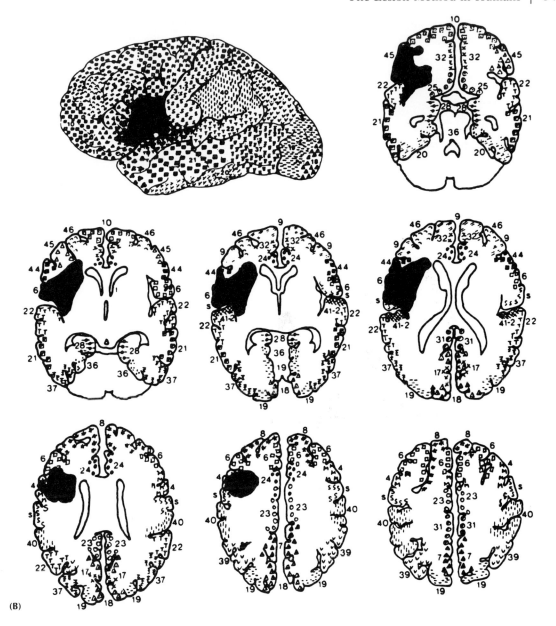

(B)

Because of its origin in mutually constraining sets of neural and cognitive data, the model is both neural and cognitive. The current version deals with neural architecture at the level of macroscopic functional regions and neuron ensembles in the primate brain. The model does not deal with microneural specifications at synaptic and molecular levels.

The cognitive architecture implicit in the model assumes (a) representations that can be described as psychological phenomena, which are interrelated according to (b) combinational semantics and com-

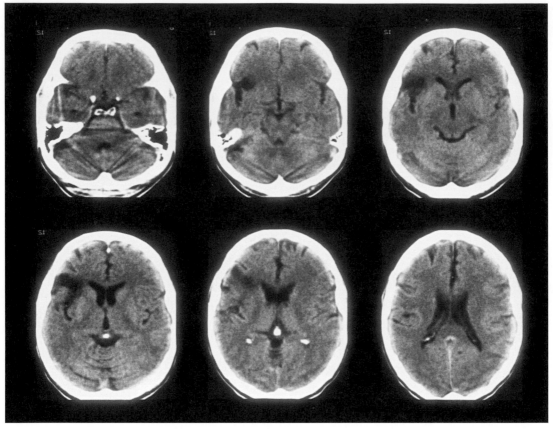

(A)

FIGURE 2.21. CT (A) and corresponding templates (B) of a 63-year-old, right-handed man who presented acutely with a marked aphasia but who regained normal speech and language within three months. Initially, this patient had labored, non-fluent speech, and had abnormal performance in most formal language tasks. His auditory comprehension was remarkably intact. Again, the overall pattern conformed to the category of Broca's aphasia, but recovery was excellent. In addition to individual differences in neural language endowment, education, and intelligence, the lesions's

binatorial syntax. The neural organization proposed here, however, is not a mere hardware implementation apparatus for *any* type of cognitive processes. Its specifications severely restrict the range of representations and algorithms that it can implement, that is, it is not likely to implement representations other than the ones its anatomy and physiology embody and are destined to operate.

The model describes an adult neural/cognitive organization it assumes to be relatively stable and yet modifiable by experience, that is, capable of temporary or stable partial reorganization. The issue of neural and cognitive development is not directly addressed, although the model does incorporate developmental assumptions.

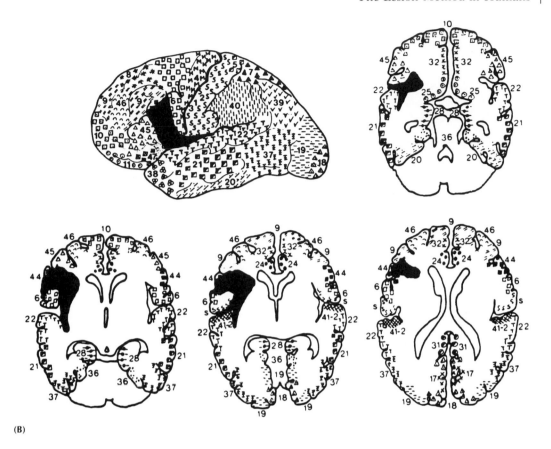

(B)

precise location is likely to play a key role in the major differences noted in the cases in Figures 2.18, 2.19 and 2.20. The extent of involvement in left dorsolateral cortices, subjacent white matter, and left basal ganglia are critical factors in the profile and outcome of these aphasias.

The chronic CT shows a well-defined area of low density limited to the most posterior portion of the left frontal operculum, with extension into the anterior portion of the insula.

The model is governed by two overall sets of constraints. The first, the *neurobiological constraints*, corresponds to the basic structural design of the nervous system and to the neuroanatomically embodied values of the organism prior to interactions with the environment. The second set, the *reality constraints*, corresponds to the characteristics of physical structure, operation, frequency of occurrence of entities and events external to the perceiver's entire organism, and of entities and events external to the perceiver's brain but internal to the body, i.e., somatic. During perceptual interactions between the perceiver's brain and its surround, the two sets of constraints lead to:

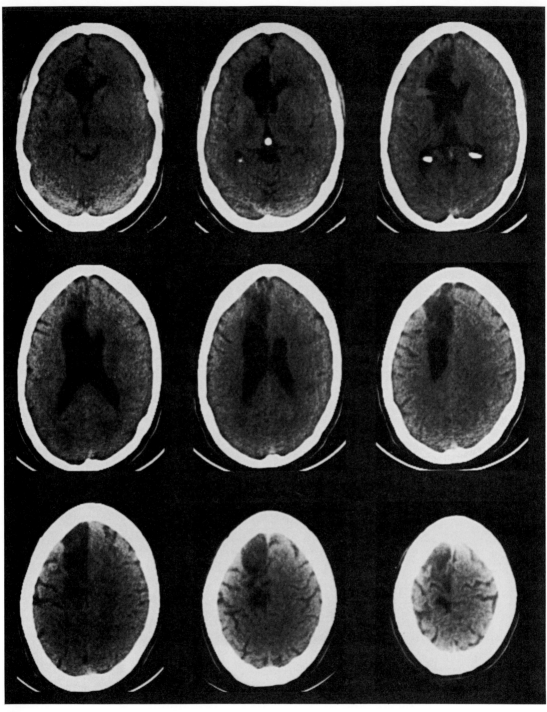

(A)

FIGURE 2.22. CT (A) and corresponding templates (B) of a 40-year-old, right-handed man. Five years earlier, he had a subarachnoid hemorrhage secondary to rupture of an anterior communicating aneurysm. This was complicated by spasm of the anterior cerebral artery and infarction in the me- sial frontal lobe. Acutely, the patient was akinetic and mute. He made no attempt to communicate by speech or gesture. Over a two-week period, he gradually began to communicate with short but grammatically correct sentences.

Three months later, he had improved markedly,

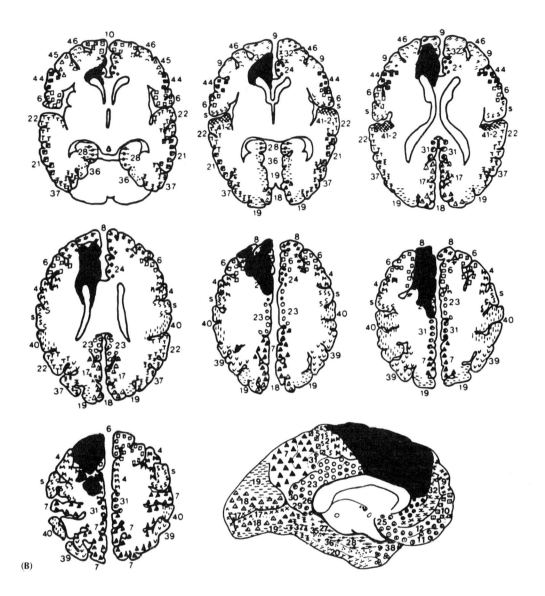

(B)

although his speech still had a nonfluent character (sentences of up to six to eight words only). Grammar was properly used. He could repeat sentences normally. Formal language testing revealed no abnormality except for his inability to generate word lists from initial letters. At the time this CT was obtained, his speech had become fluent and was nonparaphasic.

This intriguing clinical presentation, a frequent consequence of infarctions in the territory of the anterior cerebral artery, is best described as mutism with akinesia. The label transcortical motor aphasia is not appropriate because language processing *per se* is not impaired. Rather, the impairment resides with the will to communicate, by speech or gesture, and with the baseline motor routines that normally accompany an inclination to interact with the environment.

The CT shows a well-defined area of low density in the mesial aspect of the left frontal lobe involving cortex and underlying white matter. The area involved includes the anterior cingulate gyrus and mesial portion of the pre-motor area 6 (or supplementary motor area), and it extends both into the prefrontal region (area 8) and into the anterior part of the mesial motor cortex. All of the frontal lobe's dorsolateral aspect is intact.

1. *Domain formation* A process of categorization of entities and events organized on the basis of the *similarity* of physical structure, operation, frequency of occurrence, and value to the perceiver.
2. *Setting of taxomonic levels* The levels depend on the contextual complexity ranking of the perceptuo-motor activity between perceiver and entities and events.
3. *Functional regionalization* A process of assigning fragmented records of perceptuo-motor interactions, as well as of the codes binding their coincidence in time and space, to different regions of brain structure, according to domain and taxonomic level of entities and events).

The fundamental cognitive structures of the model are: (a) records of fragments of perceptual and motor events that preserve topographic/topologic relationships (*modal* sense and action data), and (b) *amodal* records of the codes that bind the occurrence of the above representations in temporal and spatial terms (*convergence zones*). The representations embodied in those structures are interrelated according to combinatorial semantics and syntax.

The neuroanatomical substrates for the above cognitive structures are:

1. Primary and early association cortices, both sensory and motor, which constitute the substrate for topographic/topologic records.
2. Association cortices of different orders, both sensory and motor, some limbic structures (entorhinal cortex, hippocampus, amygdala, cingulate cortices), the neostriatum, and the cerebellum, which constitute the substrate for binding code records.
3. Feed-forward and feedback connectivity interrelating (1) and (2).
4. Servosystem structures in thalamus, basal forebrain, hypothalamus, and brain stem nuclei.

This cognitive/neural architecture can (1) perform perceptuomotor interactions with the brain's surround; (2) learn those interactions; (3) solve problems, make decisions, plan, and create; and (4) communicate with the environment. All of those functions depend on a fundamental operation: *The attempted reconstitution of learned perceptuomotor interactions in the form of internal recall and motor performance.* This is achieved by the *retroactivation* of fragmentary records in *multiple cortical regions* as a result of feedback activity from convergence zones. According to this model, there is no single site for integrating sensory and motor processes. Spatial and temporal integration is an illusion brought about by time-locked occurrence during perception or co-evocation during recall.

Although the notion of representation covers all the inscriptions related to an entity or event, that is, a combination of fragment and binding-code records, the model posits that only the multiregional retroactivations of the fragment components can become a content of consciousness. The perceptuomotor reconstitutions that form the substrate of consciousness thus occur in an anatomically restricted sector of the brain, albeit in a distributed, multiple-site manner. Furthermore, the model posits the need for attention, which is defined on the basis of a critical level of activity in order for retroactivated fragments to become conscious.

According to this model, and unlike traditional neurological models, there is no localizable, single store for the meaning of a given stimulus within a cortical region. Meaning is arrived at by widespread multiregional activation of fragmentary records pertinent to a stimulus, wherever such records may be stored, in distributed manner, within a large array of sensory and motor structures. A display of the meaning of a stimulus does not exist in permanent fashion; it is recreated instead for each and every instantiation. The same stimulus does not produce the same evocations every time it is presented, although many of the same or similar sets of records will be evoked by the same or comparable stimuli. The records that pertain to a given entity are distributed in the telencephalon, both in the sense that they are inscribed over sizable neuron populations and in the sense that they are to be found in multiple loci of cerebral cortex and subcortical nuclei.

Background

The notion of separating storage of fragments of experience from storage of a "catalogue" for their reconstruction, arose directly from the lesion studies and especially from the study of amnesic patients. The same can be said of the notion that a unidirectional caudal-rostral processing cascade was less likely than a multidirectional, recursive organization. The specific notion of convergence zones came from reflection on neuroanatomical patterns of cortico-limbic projections. The multiplicity of parallel and converging channels, and the fact that the size of the neural convergence sites was progressively reduced along a caudal-rostral axis, were compelling. The patterned disruption of cortico-limbic and cortico-cortical feed-forward and feedback projections that we have been observing in patients with Alzheimer's disease (see Van Hoesen & Damasio, 1987, for review) provided the blueprint for the notion of convergence zone.

The notion that categorization and the building of so-called generic memories "precede" the building of episodic memories, and are, respectively, linked to caudal cortices and rostral cortices, came directly from our studies of agnosic and amnesic patients, especially subjects EH and Boswell. As will be noted in the following paragraphs, categorization occurs naturally, on the basis of feature/dimension overlap relative to multiple exemplars. The process of individualization of exemplars (that is, the process of rendering them unique and "episodic"), depends on added linkages to disambiguating mappings that occur, anatomically and functionally, downstream in the network and later in time. To our knowledge, this notion has not been advanced previously.

The notion that the perceiver's somatic states are represented according to the same rules that apply to external entities, and the importance accorded to mapping such somatic states concurrently with the mapping of external entities, are critical concepts in the model. Their source is, again, our studies of humans with focal lesions, especially those with conditions such as anosognosia and acquired conduct disorders. We are not aware of any precedent for this notion.

The concept for the operation of convergence zones was influenced by the work of Triesman on the subject of attention (Triesman & Gelade, 1980). Our conceptualization of co-attended co-activations for complex memories can be seen as a modification and extension, at a higher level of processing, of a notion first advanced by Triesman regarding the need to create some form of "conjunction" of separately processed microdimensions and features of stimuli. Notable differences include the fact that our conjunctions operate on internally generated as well as externally stimulated representational neural activity, and that there is a staggeringly large number of conjoined components for the kind of complex memories of entities and events that we propose are processed according to such principles. Francis Crick's related hypothesis for a neural device capable of selective attention was also influential (Crick, 1984).

The notion that conscious recall depends on topographical/topological activtaions, is based on introspective data. It posits that recalled experiences are based, immediately or remotely, on the activation of geometry-based components of representations.

The model provides a framework for the reinterpretation of the principal types of higher cognitive disorder—the agnosias, the amnesias, and the aphasias—and prompts new hypotheses for further investigation on the neural basis of human cognition.

Rationale

Sensory and motor patterns of neural activity constitute the base ingredients of perception and recall, regardless of how one conceptualizes the microneural structure and organization underlying the recording of experiences. Once such patterns occur (as a result of interactions between the central nervous system and the environment, as in perception, or as a result of internally triggered processes, as in recall), the physiological definition of their occurrence can be stored in relatively stable, although modifiable, manner. Later, the original neural patterns or some approximation or variation thereof can be reactivated phasically.

As noted in the previous section, evidence from both lesion studies in humans and animals, and neurophysiological studies in animals, indicates that the brain mapping of sensory and motor representations is parcelated (A. Damasio, 1985a; Ungerleider & Mishkin, 1982; Van Essen & Maunsell, 1983). Not only does a splitting of the integrated multimodal environment by sensory modality occur (that is, the mapping of an entity defined by three sensory modalities *must* occur in three separate modal channels) but, within each sensory modality, the various characteristics that define entities (features, dimensions, spatial integration of features, position of the entity space) are processed by different functional regions of a single modality cortex (Hubel & Livingstone, 1987; Mountcastle, Lynch, & Georgopoulos, 1984). Evidence from cognitive psychology studies in normal humans supports the same view (Posner, 1980; Triesman & Gelade, 1980). The condition faced by sensory and motor representations is a fragmentation of the mapping of physical reality at every scale. The physical structure of an entity, be it an external entity such as an object, or an internal entity such as a specific somatic state, is mapped in terms of separate constituent ingredients. Each ingredient is the consequence of secondary mappings at a lower physical scale. Naturally, the fragmentation is even more marked for events and abstract entities. Events are based on an interplay of entities, and abstract entities correspond to criterion-governed conjunctions of dimensions and features present in concrete entities.

As a consequence of neuroanatomical design, the components that make up the integrated, multimodal sensory experiences that represent reality's transactions occur in brain sectors that are anatomically distinct and geographically apart. Furthermore, there is neuropsychological evidence that the properties and typical operations that characterize a given entity in the environment are also processed in separate regions (see A. Damasio, H. Damasio, & Tranel, 1988). Finally, if perceptual experience is based on neural fragmentation, its recording in neurons must also be fragmented.

The central problem for the notion of perceptual or recalled representation can be stated as follows: the fact that our sensory experiences, single or multimodal, are "coherent" and "in register," at the multiple levels of the reality that the brain detects, indicates that there is an *integrative* operation capable of bringing together multiple brain activity fragments within a sensory modality and across sensory modalities. Without such multiple level and multiple modality integration, it would not be possible to generate coherent experience. Given the potential for recall and recognition of any coherently perceived experience, it is apparent that some aspects of the multiple level integration can be stored, at least in part, in relatively stable manner and over considerable periods of time.

The problem's solution must reside with brain devices capable of promoting the integration of fragmentary components of neural activity. The results of experimental neuroanatomy, neurophysiology, and the most apparent consequences of differently located cerebral lesions in humans and monkeys have led to the view that reality is progressively represented in the brain along a unidirectional cascade of sequential neural analyzers that allows for gradually more detailed extraction of stimuli's physical properties and the spatial relationships among stimuli. Two of the most influential models of higher cognitive activity in the post-war period, Geschwind's (1965) and Luria's (1966), assume this form of caudal-rostral increment of perceptual detail, which builds up towards a higher integrative level of representation, the basis for self-consciousness and executive control. To some extent, a critical body of neurophysiological and neuroanatomical discoveries have given apparent support for these views. For instance, the visual system *does* possess a chain of hierarchical analyzers that perform differently in relation to the images that impinge upon the eye. The entire visual world projects onto the retinas two-dimensional matrix and progressively generates activity in a series of processors in the lateral geniculate nuclei, the primary visual cortex, and the visual association cortices. The more peripheral the station, the more primitive is the analysis of the signals, and the more scrambled and jumbled the portrayal of reality appears to be. At the level of the visual association cortices and beyond, the analysis becomes finer and the representations richer. Higher-order association cortices receive the product of information processing in the previous stations, and the representations contained there are not only finer in detail but also polymodal, that is, data from other modalities are not conjoined in the same regions (Bruce et al, 1981; Desimone et al, 1984; Perrett, Rolls, & Caan, 1982). Further anteriorly, in this caudal-rostral progression, the entire multimodal world seems to converge in the entorhinal cortex and the hippocampal formation (Van Hoesne, 1982). Along a different but parallel route, data from multiple sensory sources also reach integration points within the prefrontal cortices (Jones & Powell, 1970; Nauta, 1971; Pandya & Kuypers, 1969). We are aware of only one exception to the dominant view of anterior cerebral structures as the end of the processing cascade (in the work of Crick, 1984, related to a hypothesis for a neural mechanisms underlying attention).

The several integrative neuroanatomical units of the anterior temporal cortices, medial temporal limbic system, and prefrontal cortices have provided a superficially satisfactory solution to the fragmentation problem, because of their potential to bring sense data together. Our view, however, is that this solution is *not* satisfactory. We question the existence of unidirectional cascade, even if it is conceived as parallel, rather than single and sequential. We also question the information processing mataphor implicit in such models. Our principal objection, however, comes from the fact that if rostral integrative units are the answer to fragmentation, then the results of their selective damage in human experiments reveal a troubling paradox.

THE CENTRAL PARADOX

If the full integration of neural activity on the basis of which the experience of representations unfolds occurs in anterior temporal and frontal integrative units, the following predictions should be verified:

1. Bilateral destruction of those units precludes the perception of reality as a coherent multimodal experience and reduces experience to modal tracks of sensory or motor processing.
2. Bilateral destruction of integrative units reduces the quality of even such modal track processing, for example, reduces the richness and detail of perception commensurate with the quality obtainable by the level of perceptual stations left intact.
3. Bilateral damage to integrative units entails the destruction of the memory records of the entire past experience, for all levels and types of memory, that is, (a) memory for specific entities and events, including those that constitute the perceiver's autobiography, (b) memory for specific but nonunique entities and events, and (c) memory for relationships among events, entities, and features of entities and events.

However, reflection on the results of bilateral destruction of the anterior temporal regions, as well as bilateral destruction of prefrontal cortices, either in separate sectors or in combination, denies all but a fraction of one of these predictions.

THE EVIDENCE

It is *not* true that bilateral lesions of the temporal integrative units prevent coherent, multimodal, perceptual experience. It is *not* true that those lesions cause a diminution of experience's perceptual quality. On the contrary, all available experimental neuropsychological evidence indicates that the quality of perceptual experience of subjects who have sustained major selective damage to their anterior temporal lobes is comparable to controls (Corkin, 1984; A.

Damasio et al, 1985a; A. Damasio et al, 1987). Those subjects report on what they see, hear, and touch in ways that observers cannot distinguish from what they themselves report. Covert knowledge paradigms, such as forced recognition, and passive skin conductance reveal that they can also discriminate stimuli in a manner that indicates a rich nonconscious activation of perceptual detail (Tranel & A. Damasio, 1985, 1986, 1987, to be published). The nonautobiographical knowledge that such subjects can consciously evoke about the world indicates that vast "integrated" memory stores have not been compromised by damage to the alleged integrative units.

The only accurate prediction regarding the role of the temporal integrative units, pertains to the loss of the ability to evoke unique combinations of representations that were conjoined in experience within specific time and space units. That ability is indeed lost, and so is the possibility of creating records for such new experiences. This is best demonstrated by the neuropsychological profile of our subject, Boswell, whose cerebral damage entirely destroyed, bilaterally, both hippocampal systems (including the entorhinal cortex, the hippocampal formation, and the amygdala), the cortices in anterolateral and anteroinferior temporal lobes (including those in areas 38, 20, 21, anterior sector of 22, and part of 37), the entire basal forebrain region bilaterally, and the most posterior part of the orbitofrontal cortices, also bilaterally (see Figure 2.13). Boswell has intact perception in all modalities but the olfactory. The descriptions he produces of complex visual or auditory entities and events are indistinguishable from those of his examiners. All aspects of his motor performance are perfect. His memory for most external entities is preserved, at the generic/categorical level. A memory defect only becomes evident when subordinate taxonomic specificity is required, that is, the recognition of uniqueness. Also intact are grammar, phonemic and phonetic processing, and prosody. In brief, Boswell's perceptuo-motor interaction with the environment remains intact, provided specificity of perception or action is not required. Multimodal recognition, recall, and imagery operate capably for large sectors of generic/categorical knowledge.

Damage to the integrative units in bilateral prefrontal cortices, whether restricted to the orbitofrontal sector, the dorsolateral sector, or the entire prefrontal regions, is entirely compatible with normal perceptual processes and even with normal memory for entities and events. The only exception is the domain of complex social knowledge. Evidence includes Brickner's patient A, and the patients of Hebb, and Ackerly and Benton (see A. Damasio, 1985b, for review), as well as our subject, EVR (Eslinger & Damasio, 1985). The frontal lobe structures, with their multiple and relatively independent sites for the termination of processing cascades, are unlikely candidates for a comprehensive integration, even less so than their temporal counterparts (A. Damasio, 1979). At best, frontal lobe structures can be viewed as "guides" and "teachers" of posteriorly located circuitry, rather than as the culmination of cerebral physiology (A. Damasio, 1979).

Perhaps even more paradoxical is the fact that damage within certain sectors of sensory association cortices does affect quality of perception and always within a single modality (A. Damasio, 1985a; A. Damasio et al, 1982b). Damage within modal sensory association cortices can disturb recall and recognition of stimuli presented through that modality. *Any* domain of stimuli, at *any* taxonomic level, can be disturbed, depending on the specification of the lesion in terms of functional region placement, size, and uni- or bi-laterality. Lesions within visual association cortices may impair the recognition of the unique identity of faces but allow for the recognition of facial expressions, nonunique objects, and visual-verbal material. Or they may compromise object recognition and leave face recognition intact, or compromise reading but not object or face recognition. The important fact is that damage in a caudal and modal association cortex *can disrupt recall and recognition at the most subordinate taxonomic level,* that of uniqueness, and so preclude the kind of integrated experience usually associated in theory with the rostral cortices. Lesions in modal cortices also reduce the potential for modality-based imagery (Farah, to be published), and disrupt learning of new entities and events presented through the modality (A. Damasio, H. Damasio, & Tranel, 1988).

Another Solution

The consideration of the previous evidence and of additional neuropsychological and neuroanatomical findings in humans has led us to the formulation of a neural organization model in which:

1. The activity that embodies the perceptual representations of *the physical structure of any entity must occur in fragmented fashion and in geographically separate cortices* located in (a) the modal sensory cortices usually referred to as "early," "posterior," and "caudal," and the (b) precentral motor cortices. The so-called "integrative," "rostral" cortices of the anterior temporal and prefrontal regions do *not* contain the inscription of the finest representations necessary for integrated experience.

2. The integration of multiple aspects of external and internal reality in perceptual or recalled experiences, both within each modality and across modalities, depends on the *co-activation or geographically separate sites of neural activity* within *sensory and motor cortices,* rather than on a neural transfer and integration of different representations towards rostral neural integration sites.

3. The patterns of neural activity that describe physical structure fragments can be recorded in the neural ensembles in which they occur during perception, but the binding codes that describe their linkages in entities and events, that is, their temporal and spatial coincidences, are stored in separate neural ensembles (convergence zones). The reactivation of physical structure fragments on which recall of experiences depends is *not* possible without the concerted operation of the neural ensembles that contain binding codes, that is, is not possible within retroactivation brought about by activity in convergence units.

4. The conscious experience of co-activations depends on their simultaneous enhancement *(co-attention)*, against the background activity on which other activations are being played back, that is, on the creation of temporary conjunctions by salience of activity.

5. The richness of the reconstruction is probability-governed. It depends not only on all the factors that affect storage but also on parameters of the stimulus and the state of the perceiver.

Taking into account other evidence from neuroanatomy, neurophysiology, and neuropsychology discussed in the following section, the model further specifies that:

1. The mechanisms for the concerted co-activation of neural activity patterns that occurred simultaneously in previous experience (or are otherwise pertinently linked) depends on activity in convergence zones located at multiple neural levels (association cortices, limbic system, subcortical nuclei). Convergence zones bind and subtend gradually larger sets of experientially conjoined sites. Cortical convergence zones are placed in *progressively more rostral and higher-order association cortices,* the larger the set of sites they conjoin. Local convergence zones bind regions, within the same modality, in which features of a given entity has been inscribed; progressively higher-order convergence zones bind wider multimodal sets of regions and are placed relatively more rostrally. There is a spatial ordering of convergence units by complexity, although there is not a linear spatial hierarchy. In other words, there is not a rigid stacking of units along neat cascades.

Convergence zones are made up of neuron ensembles that have been projected upon by multiple sensory and motor cortices in such a way that they have been informed of the co-occurrence of activation in the feeding cortices by feed-forward projections. By means of reciprocating feedback projections, convergence zones can trigger activity in all or part of the originally feeding cortices, in retroactive divergent manner, whenever one or more of its feed-forward projections activates it. Convergence units are *a*modal, in that they receive signals from the same or different modalities, but do not inscribe sensory or motor activity in a way that preserves geometry-based, topographic, and topological relations as they occured in perception. Convergence zones do not embody a refined representation, in the sense that would be assumed in an information processing model, although they do route information in the sense of information theory. They are not informed about the content of the representations they assist in reconstructing.

2. Convergence zones contain binding codes for many entities and events. Such rich binding is the source of the widening retroactivation that permits recognition, but, if unconstrained, its wealth would eventually result in co-activations bearing little relationship to previous specific experience, and ultimately being unable to reconstitute unique events. In the model, the constraints that impose specificity of co-evocations operate on the basis of *indirect influence on the convergence zone itself* and *on both feeding and subsequent stations*, from the following systems:

   a. Other convergence zones, at multiple neural levels, whose subtended retroactivation provides neural context and thus helps constrain coactivation. This includes not only convergence zones in other association cortices and in hippocampus/amygdala, but also in (i) thalamic nuclei, acting directly, by means of cortico-thalamic and thalamo-cortical projections modulated by activity in reticular nucleus; indirectly through the action of anterior, dorsomedial, and medial nonspecific nuclei, over the hippocampus and amygdala, prefrontal cortices, and anterior cingulate cortices; (ii) basal ganglia (from the caudate nucleus via the pallidum, the motor thalamus, the supplementary motor area, and the lateral aspect of area 6; also via the substantia nigra to dorsomedial thalamus and prefrontal cortex); (iii) cerebellum (via the motor thalamus and motor cortices);

   b. Nonspecific limbic nuclei (basal forebrain and brain stem) activated by antero-temporal limbic units (amygdala, hippocampus).

3. The temporal locking of activities in multiple sites that is necessary for temporary conjunctions is achieved by iteration across time phases.

In brief, the model proposes not a single direction of processing, along a single channel, but rather a *parallel, convergent, and divergent, nonlinear, recursive,* and *iterative* form of processing. Convergence zones provide integration, and although the convergence zones that realize the more encompassing integration are indeed more rostrally placed, the activity that all levels of convergence zone promote, and on the basis of which representations are reconstructed and evoked, actually takes place in "caudal" rather than "rostral" cortices. The sensory and motor cortices are the sector of the brain on which *both* perception and recall play themselves out, and on which self-consciousness must necessarily be based.

ADDITIONAL EVIDENCE

Current knowledge from neurophysiology and neuroanatomy indicates that the proposed solution is indeed possible. For instance, evidence exists for separate and parallel streams of sensory processing within the visual system. Hubel and Livingstone (Hubel & Livingstone, 1987; Livingstone & Hubel, 1984) have shown that different columns within area 17 are dedicated to the processing of color and of different aspects of form. Beyond area 17, the anatomical and functional organization can be described as follows:

1. Evidence exists for early channel separation and divergence into a multitude of functional regions; this has been revealed by neurophysiological studies (Allman et al, 1985; Van Essen & Maunsell, 1983), and characterized in part by studies of neuroanatomical connectivity (Gilbert, 1983; Lund et al, 1981; Rockland & Pandya, 1979, 1981; Zeki, personal communication, 1979); the organization is describable by the attributes *divergent, one-to-many, parallel,* and *sequential.*

2. Evidence exists for back-projections to the feeding origin, capable of affecting processing in a *retroactive* manner, and of cross-projections to maps of the same level (Van Essen, 1985).

3. Evidence exists for convergence into functional regions downstream. Projections from visual, auditory, and somatosensory cortices can be encountered in combinations from bimodal or trimodal sources, in progressively more rostral brain regions, such as areas 37, 36, 38, 21 and 20 (Jones & Powell, 1970; Seltzer & Pandya, 1976; Van Hoesen, personal communication, 1988). This design feature is describable by the attributes *convergent, many-to-few, parallel,* and *sequential.* (In humans, judging from evidence in nonhuman primates, trimodal integration is likely to take place in functional regions within Brodmann's areas 36, 37, 38, 39.).

4. Evidence exists for continued retrodivergence from the latter cortices, which are also equipped with feedback, that is, convergence regions have the power to back-project in divergent manner to the feeding cortices.

5. The pattern of forward convergence and retrodivergence is again repeated in the rostral cerebral cortices of the entorhinal and prefrontal regions. In both, neuron ensembles that have received convergent projections from neurons located in multimodal cortices can project into yet smaller neuron groups, as in layer II and the superficial part of layer III of the entorhinal cortex (Van Hoesen, 1982). We describe this feature of cerebral design as *convergent* and *few-to-fewer.* The influence of this convergence activity is felt in the

hippocampal formation proper, by means of the perforant pathway projections to the dentate gyrus and of projections from there into the ammonic field sequence of CA4, CA3, and CA1. Once again, convergence is followed by a pattern of divergent feedback, which uses several anatomical routes: (a) a direct route, using the subiculum and layer IV of the entorhinal cortex, diverges into the cortices that provide the last station of input into hippocampus (Van Hoesen, 1982). As noted previously, those cortices can, in turn, project back to the previous feeding station; (b) an indirect route, so far only revealed in rodents but possibly present in primates as well, which can feedback into virtually all previous stations, divergently and in saltatory fashion, rather than in recapitulatory manner (Swanson & Kohler, 1986); and (c) an even less direct and specific route, which uses pathways in the fornix and exerts influence over thalamic, hypothalamic, basal forebrain, and frontal structures, all of which, in turn, directly and indirectly, can influence the operation of the cerebral cortices in widespread fashion. The latter route constitutes a servosystem of back-projections that provide the cortex with regionally selective or widespread neurochemical influence (for example, acetylcholine, noradrenaline, etc.) based on the activity of neurotransmitter nuclei in the basal forebrain and brainstem.

Situating the Model

The model described above deals, in joint fashion, with cognitive and neural phenomena at the level of systems organization. To define its relative position, we will refer to two models of cognitive and neural organization: a "classical" model of cognitive architecture, as presented by Fodor & Pylyshyn (1988), and a set of models known under the designations of "connectionism" or parallel distributed processing (see Rumelhart & McClelland, 1986, McClelland & Rumelhart 1986).

Our model occupies an intermediate position. The ogranization we propose can implement some predicates of a classical cognitive architecture, while it is conceivable that connectionist nets and algorithms may be a way to realize the microscopic aspects of the organization proposed here. The model is also compatible with neuron group selection theory (Edelman & Finkel, 1984). Our view is that connectionism and neuron group selection are, primarily, theories of neural microstructure rather than models for neural nets capable of higher cognition. Although the "neuron units" in those models share some characteristics of real neurons, the networks are not yet "brain-like." More importantly, the principles of structure and operation of the machines so designed do not predict the higher order organization necessary for processes such as episodic memory, thought, language, or consciousness, that is, they do not compel separate components to hook up in such a way that would make the system thoughtful and self-conscious.

We believe this model contains several novel features. The most salient are as follows:

1. The value accorded to representations of internal somatic states. Somatic states have the same status given to representations of external entities. External entities and events are always recorded along with the co-occurring somatic state, and consequently, reality is inscribed as an interaction with the perceiver's organism.

Somatic states are often relegated to a subsidiary position, a nonspecific influence on the operation of a network concerned with representing external reality. In this model, somatic states are entitled to geometry-based, topographically or topologically organized evocable fragments, as well as to binding convergence zones.

2. The distinction between (a) *records of physical structure fragments*, and (b) *records of binding codes for relations* among physical structure records.

The former (i) are feature-based; (ii) are analog; (iii) are distributed within "early" sensory modal cortices and "late" motor cortices; (iv) can be played back phasically by retroactivation as a result of reencounter with original stimulus or internally generated recall.

The latter (i) are *a*modal; (ii) do not preserve reality-like topographic or topologic relationships; (iii) are located in convergence zones within association cortices of different orders, hippocampus, thalamus, basal ganglia, and cerebellum. They are the sole key to the binding of fragmentary records.

This view is different from the traditional neurological notion of "image" representations, and from the notion of representation implicit in connectionist models and neuron group selection theory. In those models there are no geometry-based components to representations, which are, instead, incribed in purely *a*modal fashion throughout the network.

3. The notion that the experience of entities or events in recall (the generation of evocations) always depends on retroactivation of fragmentary records contained in multiple sensory and motor regions and thus on momentary reconstructions of the once perceived components of representations of reality.

4. The notion that although evocations only exist momentarily, they are nevertheless the only directly inspectable aspect of cognition. Their fleeting existence makes them no less real. Furthermore, although their existence depends on a complex machinery distributed by multiple brain sites and levels, the model specifies that *the reconstructions themselves occur in an anatomically restricted sector of the cerebrum*, albeit in a distributed, multiple site manner.

5. The notion of co-attention as a means to transform covert activations into experienceable representational contents (evocations).

6. The value attributed to feedback projections, especially cortico-cortical, as part of the anatomical substrate for the mechanisms of reconstitution of experiences. (Feedback is different from re-entry as used in the automata of Edelman and Reeke (1982). Both feedback and feedforward carry signals "about" activity in interconnected units but they do not "transport" a moving representation being "entered" or "re-entered." Feed-forward signals mark the presence of activity upstream in the network and generally indicate provenance. Feedback reactivates records located upstream. The convergence zone records relationships "abstractly" and merely operates to direct activity. The early representations of reality are not transferred in the system, that is, no concrete contents and no information in the psychological sense move about in the system.)

7. The notion that certain aspects of the interaction between perceiver and reality, such as (a) the similarity of physical structure, (b) the similarity of operation, (c) the similarity of somatic states accompanying perception, (d) the taxonomic level of the entity or event in absolute terms as well as in the perceiver's biographic perspective and species value system, contribute to generate domains of knowledge.

References

Alexander MP, Freeman M: Amnesia after anterior communicating artery aneurysm rupture. *Neurology* **33**(suppl 2):104, 1983.

Alexander MP, Schmitt MA: The aphasia syndrome of stroke in the left anterior cerebral artery territory. *Archives of Neurology* **37**:97–100, 1980.

Allman J, Miezin F. McGuinnes E: Stimulus specific responses from beyond the classical receptive field: Neuropsychological mechanisms for local-global comparisons in visual neurons. In *Annual Review of Neuroscience*, vol. 8, pp 407–430, 1985.

Anderson S, Tranel D: Unawareness of cognitive and motor deficits: Neuropsychologic and neuroanatomic factors. *Journal of Clinical and Experimental Neuropsychology* **10**(1):24, 1988.

Aran DM, Rose DF, Rekate HL, Whitaker HA: Acquired capsular/striatal aphasia in childhood. *Archives of Neurology* **40**:614–617, 1983.

Balint R: Seelenlähmung des "Schauens," optische Ataxie, räumliche Störung der Aufmerksamkeit. *Monatsschrift der Psychiatrie und Neurologie* **25**:51–81, 1909.

Bellugi U, Poizner H, Klima ES: Sign language aphasia. *Human Neurobiology* **2**:155–170, 1983.

Benson DF, Sheremata WA, Bouchard R, Segarra JM, Price DL, Geschwind N: Conduction aphasia: A clinicopathological study. *Archives of Neurology* **28**:339–346, 1973.

Benton A, Hamsher K, Varney AR, Spreen O: *Contributions to Neuropsychological Assessment.* New York, Oxford University Press, 1983.

Blumstein SE: *A Phonological Investigation of Aphasia Speech.* Mouton, The Hague, 1978.

Bouillaud JB: Recherches cliniques propres à démontrer que la perte de la parole correspond à la lésion des lobules anterieurs du cerveau. *Archives Générales de Medicine* **8:**24–45, 1825.

Bradley DC, Garrett ME, Zurif EB: Syntactic deficits in Broca's aphasia. In Caplan D (ed): *Biological Studies of Mental Processes.* Cambridge, MA, MIT Press, 1980.

Broca P: Localisation des fonctions cérébrales: Siège du langage articulé. *Bulletin de la Société d'Anthropologie* **4:**200–203, 1863.

Broca P: Du siège de la faculté du langage articulé. *Bulletin de la Société d'Anthropologie* **6:**337–393, 1865.

Bruce C, Desimone R, Gross CG: Visual properties of neurons in a polysensory area in superior temporal sulcus of the macaque. *Journal of Neurophysiology* **46:**369–384, 1981.

Brunner RJ, Kornhuber HH, Seemuller E, Suger G, Wallesch CW: Basal ganglia participation in language pathology. *Brain and Language* **16:**281–299, 1982.

Caplan D, Futter F: Assignment of thematic roles to nouns in sentence comprehension by an agrammatic patient. *Brain and Language* **27:**117–134, 1986.

Caramazza A, Zurif EG: Dissociation of algorithmic and heuristic processes in language comprehension: Evidence from aphasia. *Brain and Language* **3:**572–582, 1976.

Cohen NJ, Squire LR: Preserved learning and retention of pattern-analyzing skill in amnesia: Dissociation of knowing how and knowing that. *Science* **210:**207–210, 1980.

Corkin S: Lasting consequences of bilateral medial temporal lobectomy: Clinical course and experimental findings in HM. *Seminars in Neurology* **4:**249–259, 1984.

Cowan WM: Neuronal death as a regulative mechanism in the control of cell number in the nervous system. In Rockskin M, Sussman M (eds): *Development and Aging in the Nervous System,* pp 19–41. New York, Academic Press, 1973.

Cowan WM, Fawcett JW, O'Leary D, Stanfield B: Regressive events in neurogenesis. *Science* **225:**1258–1265, 1984.

Crick F: Function of the thalamic reticular complex: The searchlight hypothesis. *Proceedings at the National Academy of Science* **81:**4586–4590, 1984.

Damasio A: The frontal lobes. In Heilman K, Valenstein E (eds): *Clinical Neuropsychology,* ed 1, pp 360–412. New York, Oxford University Press, 1979.

Damasio A: Language and the basal ganglia. *Trends in Neuroscience* **6:**442–443, 1983.

Damasio A: Disorders of complex visual processing. In *Principles of Behavioral Neurology, Contemporary Neurology Series,* pp 259–288. Philadelphia, F. A. Davis, 1985a.

Damasio A: The frontal lobes. In: Heilman K, Valenstein E (eds): *Clinical Neuropsychology,* ed 2. New York, Oxford University Press, 1985b.

Damasio A: Language and the basal ganglia. In Evarts EV, Wise SP, Bousfield D (eds): *The Motor System in Neurobiology,* pp 288–291. Amsterdam, Elsevier Biomedical Press, 1985c.

Damasio A: The brain binds entities and events by multiregional activation from convergence zones. *Neural Computation* **1:**123–132, 1989a.

Damasio A: Multiregional co-attended retroactivation: A new model of the neural substrates of cognition. *Cognition* 1989b.

Damasio A, Damasio H: The anatomical basis of pure alexia. *Neurology* **33**(12):1573–1583, 1983.

Damasio A, Tranel T: Domain-specific amnesia for social knowledge. *Society for Neuroscience, Abstracts* vol. 14, 1988.

Damasio A, Van Hoesen GW: Staining the human brain. *Archives of Neurology* **36:**813, 1979.

Damasio A, Van Hoesen, GW: Structure and function of the supplementary motor area. *Neurology* **30:**359, 1980.

Damasio A, Van Hoesen, GW: Emotional disturbances associated with focal lesions of the limbic frontal lobe. In Heilman K, Satz P (eds): *The Neuropsychology of Human Emotion: Recent Advances*, pp 85–110. New York, The Guilford Press, 1983.

Damasio A, Damasio H, Tranel D: Impairments of visual recognition as clues to the processes of categorization and memory. In Edelman G, Gall E, Cowan M (eds): *Signal Sense: Local and Global Order in Perceptual Maps*, Neuroscience Institute Monograph. New York, Wiley & Sons, 1989.

Damasio A, Damasio H, Van Hoesen GW: Prosopagnosia: Anatomic basis and behavioral mechanisms. *Neurology* **32:**331–341, 1982b.

Damasio A, Yamada T, Damasio H, Corbett J, McKee J: Central achromatopsia: Behavioral, anatomic and physiologic aspects. *Neurology* **30:**1064–1071, 1980.

Damasio A, Damasio H, Rizzo M, Varney N, Gersh F: Aphasia with nonhemorrhagic lesions in the basal ganglia and internal capsule. *Archives of Neurology* **39:**15–20, 1982a.

Damasio A, Eslinger P, Damasio H, Van Hoesen GW, Cornell S: Multimodal amnesic syndrome following bilateral temporal and basal forebrain damage. *Archives of Neurology* **42:**252–259, 1985a.

Damasio A, Graff-Radford N, Eslinger P, Damasio H, Kassell N: Amnesia following basal forebrain lesions. *Archives of Neurology* **42:**263–271, 1985b.

Damasio A, Bellugi U, Damasio H, Poizner H, Van Gilder J: Sign language aphasia during left hemisphere Amytal injection. *Nature* **322:**363–365, 1986.

Damasio A, Damasio H, Tranel D, Welsh K, Brandt J: Additional neural and cognitive evidence in patient DRB. *Society for Neuroscience* **13:**1452, 1987.

Damasio H: Cerebral localization of the aphasias. In Sarno MT (ed): *Acquired Aphasia*, pp 27–65. New York, Academic Press, 1981.

Damasio H: Anatomical and neuroimaging contributions to the study of aphasia. In Goodglass H (ed): *Handbook of Neuropsychology*, vol. II. Elsevier Publishers, Amsterdam, 1989.

Damasio H, Damasio A: The anatomical basis of conduction aphasia. *Brain* **103:**337–350, 1980.

Damasio H: Eslinger P, Adams HP: Aphasia following basal ganglia lesions: New evidence. *Seminars in Neurology* **4**(2):151–161, 1984.

De Renzi E: *Disorders of Space Exploration and Cognition.* New York, Wiley, 1982.

Desimone R, Albright TD, Gross CG, Bruce C: Stimulus-selective responses of inferior temporal neurons in the macaque. *Journal of Neuroscience* **4:**2051–2062, 1984.

Edelman GM, Finkel LH: Neuronal group selection in the cerebral cortex. In Edelman GM, Gall WE, Cowan WM (eds): *Dynamic Aspects of Neocortical Function*, pp 653–695. New York, Wiley & Sons, 1984.

Edelman GM, Reeke Jr GN: Selective networks capable of representative transformations, limited generalizations, and associative memory. *Proceedings of the National Academy of Science* **79:**2091–2095, 1982.

Eslinger P, Damasio A: Severe cognitive disturbance of higher cognition after bilateral frontal lobe ablation. *Neurology* **35:**1731–1741, 1985.

Eslinger P, Damasio A: Preserved motor learning in Alzheimer's disease. *Journal of Neuroscience* **6**(10):3006–3009, 1986.

Farah M: Impaired representation of space. In Damasio A (ed): *Handbook of Neuropsychology*, vol. II. Elsevier Publishers, Amsterdam, 1989.

Fodor JA, Pylyshyn ZW: Connectionism and cognitive architecture: A critical analysis. *Cognition* **28**:3–71, 1988.

Freedman M, Alexander MP, Naeser MA: Anatomic basis of transcortical motor aphasia. *Neurology* **40**:409–417, 1984.

Freud S: *On Aphasia*, New York, International University Press, 1891/1953.

Fromkin VA: The lexicon: Evidence from acquired dyslexia. *Language* **63**:1–22, 1987.

Galaburda AM, Pandya DN: The intrinsic architectonic and connectional organization of the superior temporal region of the rhesus monkey. *The Journal of Comparative Neurology* **221**:169–184, 1983.

Gardner H: *The Mind's New Science, A History of the Cognitive Revolution*. New York, Basic Books, 1985.

Gardner H, Brownell HH, Wapner W, Michelow D: Missing the point: The role of the right hemisphere in the processing of complex linguistic materials. In Pericman E (ed): *Cognitive Process and the Right Hemisphere*. New York, Academic Press, 1983.

Geschwind N: Disconnexion syndromes in animals and man. *Brain* **88**:237–294, 1965.

Gilbert CD: Microcircuitry of the visual cortex. *Annual Review of Neuroscience* **6**:217–247, 1983.

Goldberg ME, Colby CL: The neurophysiology of spatial vision. In Damasio A: (ed.), *Handbook of Neuropsychology*, section on Visual Behavior, Elsevier, Amsterdam, 1989.

Goldman-Rakic, P. S. (1988). Topography of cognition: Parallel distributed networks in primate association cortex. In: *Annual Review of Neuroscience*, Annual Reviews Inc., Palo Alto, CA. Vol II pp 137–156.

Goodglass H, Kaplan E: *The Assessment of Aphasia and Related Disorders*. Philadelphia, Lea & Febiger, 1972.

Graff-Radford N, Eslinger P, Damasio A, Yamada T: Nonhemorrhagic infarctions of the thalamus: Behavioral anatomical and physiological correlates. *Neurology* **34**(1):14–23, 1984.

Graff-Radford N, Damasio H, Yamada T, Eslinger P, Damasio A: Nonhemorrhagic thalamic infarctions: Clinical neurophysiological and electrophysiological findings in four anatomical groups defined by CT. *Brain*, **108**:485–516, 1985.

Gross CG, Rocha-Miranda CE, Bender DB: Visual properties of neurons in inferotemporal cortex of the macaque. *Journal of Neurophysiology* **35**:96–111, 1972.

Heilman KM, Watson R, Valenstein E: Neglect and related disorders. In: Heilman KM, Valenstein E (eds): *Clinical Neuropsychology*, ed 2. New York, Oxford University Press, 1985.

Holmes G: Disturbances of vision by cerebral lesions. *British Journal of Ophthalmology* **2**:353, 1918a.

Holmes G: Disturbances of visual orientation. *British Journal of Ophthalmology*, **2**:449–486, 506–516, 1918b.

Hubel DH, Livingstone MS: Segregation of form, color, and stereopsis in primate area 18. *Journal of Neuroscience* **7**:3378–3415, 1987.

Hubel DH, Wiesel TN: Functional architecture of macaque monkey visual cortex. *Proceedings of the Royal Society*, London, Series B **198**:1–59, 1977.

Hyman BT, Damasio AR, Van Hoesen GW, Barnes CL: Alzheimer's disease: Cell specific pathology isolates the hippocampal formation. *Science* **225:**1168–1170, 1984.

Jackson H: *Selected Writings of Hughlings Jackson.* New York, Basic Books, 1958.

Jones EG, Peters A (eds): *Cerebral Cortex.* New York, Plenum Press, 1986.

Jones EG, Powell TPS: An anatomical study of converging sensory pathways within the cerebral cortex of the monkey. *Brain* **93:**793–820, 1970.

Kean ML: The linguistic interpretation of aphasic syndromes: Agrammatism in Broca's aphasia, an example. *Cognition* **5:**9–46, 1977.

Kertesz A: *Aphasia and Associated Disorders.* New York, Grune & Stratton, 1979.

Konorski J, Kozniewska H, Stepien L: Analysis of symptoms and cerebral localization of audio-verbal aphasia. *Proceedings of the VII International Congress of Neurology* **2:**234–236, 1961.

Kosslyn SM: *Image and Mind.* Cambridge, MA: Harvard University Press, 1980.

Kritchevsky M, Graff-Radford NR, Damasio A: Normal memory following damage to medial thalamus. *Archives of Neurology* **44:**959–962, 1987.

Laplane D, Talairach J, Meininger V. Clinical consequences of corticectomies involving the supplementary motor area in man. *Journal of the Neurological Sciences* **34:**301–314, 1977.

Lashley K: In search of the engram. *Symposia of the Society for Experimental Biology* **4:**454–482, 1950.

Lezak MD: *Neuropsychological Assessment,* ed 2. New York, Oxford University Press, 1983.

Lichtheim L: On aphasia. *Brain* **7:**433–484, 1885.

Livingstone MS, Hubel DH: Anatomy and physiology of a color system in the primate visual cortex. *Journal of Neuroscience* **4:**309–356, 1984.

Lund JS, Hendrickson AE, Ogren MP, Tobin EA: Anatomical organization of primate visual cortex area VII. *Journal of Comparative Neurology* **202:**19–45, 1981.

Luria AR: *Higher Cortical Functions in Man.* New York, Basic Books, 1966.

Mair WGP, Warrington EK, Weiskrantz L: Memory disorders in Korsakoff's psychosis: A neuropathological and neuropsychological investigation of two cases. *Brain* **102:**749–783, 1979.

Marshall JC, Newcombe F: Patterns of paralexia: A psycholinguistic approach. *Journal of Psycholinguistics Research* **2:**175–199, 1973.

McClelland JL, Rumelhart DE: *Parallel Distributed Processing,* vol. 2. Cambridge, MA, MIT Press, 1986.

Meadows JC: Disturbed perception of colors associated with localized cerebral lesions. *Brain* **97:**615–632, 1974a.

Meadows JC: The anatomical basis of prosopagnosia. *Journal of Neurology, Neurosurgery and Psychiatry* **37:**489–501, 1974b.

Mesulam M M: Tracing neural connections of human brain with selective silver impregnation. *Archives of Neurology* **36:**814–818, 1979.

Mesulam M-M: A cortical network for directed attention and unilateral neglect. *Annals of Neurology* **10:**309, 1981.

Milner B: Amnesia following operation on the temporal lobes. In Whitty C, Zangwill O, (eds): *Traumatic Amnesia,* pp 109–133. London, Butterworth, 1966.

Milner B, Corkin S, Teuber H-L: Further analyses of the hippocampal amnesic syndrome: 14-year follow-up study of H.M. *Neuropsychologia* **6:**215–234, 1968.

Mountcastle VB, Lynch JC, Georgopoulous A: Posterior parietal association cortex of the monkey: Command functions for operations within extrapersonal space. *Journal of Neurophysiology* **38:**871–908, 1975.

Mountcastle VB, Motter BC, Steinmetz MA, Duffy CJ: Looking and seeing: The visual functions of the parietal lobe. In Edelman GM, Gall WE, Cowan WM (eds): *Dynamic Aspects of Neocortical Function,* pp 159–193. New York, Wiley, 1984.

Naeser MA, Hayward RW: Lesion localization in aphasia with cranial computed tomography and the Boston Diagnostic Aphasia Exam. *Neurology* **28:**545–551, 1978.

Naeser MA, Alexander MP, Helm-Estabrooks N, Levine HL, Laughlin SA, Geschwind N: Aphasia with predominantly subcortical lesion sites—Description of three capsular/putaminal aphasia syndromes. *Archives of Neurology* **39:**2–14, 1982.

Nauta WJH: The problem of the frontal lobe: A reinterpretation. *Journal of Psychiatric Research* **8:**167–187, 1971.

Newcombe F: *Missile Wounds of the Brain.* London, Oxford University Press, 1969.

Newcombe F, Ratcliff G: Disorders of visuospatial analysis. In Damasio A (ed): *Handbook of Neuropsychology,* vol II. Elsevier Publishers, Amsterdam, 1989.

Ojemann GA: Brain organization for language from the perspective of electrical stimulation mapping. *The Behavioral and Brain Sciences* **189:**230, 1983.

Pandya DN, Kuypers HGJM: Cortico-cortical connections in the rhesus monkey. *Brain Research* **13:**13–36, 1969.

Perrett DI, Rolls ET, Caan W: Visual neurons responsive to faces in the monkey temporal cortex. *Experimental Brain Research* **47:**329–342, 1982.

Poizner H, Klima ES, Bellugi U: *What the Hands Reveal About the Brain.* Boston, Bradford Books, 1987.

Posner MI: Orienting of attention. *Quarterly Journal of Experimental Psychology* **32:**3–25, 1980.

Purves D, Lichtman JW: Elimination of synapses in the developing nervous system. *Science* **210:**153–157, 1980.

Rakic P: Genetic and epigenetic determinants of local neuronal circuits in the mammalian central nervous system. In Schmitt FO, Worden FG (eds): *The Neurosciences: Fourth Study Program,* pp 109–127. Cambridge, MA, MIT Press, 1979.

Rakic P: Principles of neuronal migration. In Cowan WM (ed): *Handbook of Physiology: Developmental Neurobiology* Bethesda, MD, American Physiological Society, 1985.

Rizzo M, Damasio H: Impairment of stereopsis with focal brain lesions. *Annals of Neurology* **18**(1):112, 1985.

Rizzo M, Hurtig R, Damasio A: The role of scanpaths in facial recognition and learning. *Annals of Neurology* **22:**41–45, 1987.

Rockland KS, Pandya DN: Laminar origins and terminations of cortical connections of the occipital lobe in the rhesus monkey. *Brain Research* **179:**3–20, 1979.

Rockland KS, Pandya DN: Cortical connections of the occipital lobe in the rhesus monkey: Interconnections between areas 17, 18, 19 and the superior temporal gyrus. *Brain Research* **212:**249–270, 1981.

Rolls ET, Baylis GC, Leonard CM: Role of low and high spatial frequencies in the face-selective responses of neurons in the cortex in the superior temporal sulcus in the monkey. *Vision Research* **25:**1021–1035, 1985.

Rolls ET, Perrett DI, Caan W, Wilson FA: Neuronal responses related to visual recognition. *Brain* **105:**611–646, 1982.

Rosch E, Mervis C, Gray W, Johnson D, Boyes-Braem P: Basic objects in natural categories. *Cognitive Psychology* **8:**382–439, 1976.

Ross M, Damasio H, Eslinger P: The role of the supplementary motor area (SMA) and anterior cingulate (AC) in the generation of movement. *Neurology* **36**(1):346, 1986.

Rubens A, Selnes O: Aphasia with insular cortex infarction. *Proceedings of the Academy of Aphasia, 26th Meeting*. Nashville, 1986.

Rumelhart DE, McClelland JL: *Parallel Distributed Processing*, vol. 1. Cambridge, MA, MIT Press, 1986.

Saffran EM, Schwartz MF, Marin OSM: The word order problem in agrammatism. II. Production. *Brain and Language* **10**:263–280, 1980.

Schwartz MF, Marin OSM, Saffran EM: The word order problem in agrammatism I. Comprehension. *Brain and Language* **10**:249–262, 1980.

Seltzer B, Pandya DN: Some cortical projections to the parahippocampal area in the rhesus monkey. *Experimental Neurology* **50**:146–160, 1976.

Shepard RN, Cooper LA: *Mental Images and Their Transformations*. Cambridge, MA, MIT Press, 1982.

Sperry RW: Cerebral organization and behavior. *Science* **133**:1749–1757, 1961.

Squire LR, Amaral DG, Zola-Morgan S, Kritchevsky M, Press G: New evidence of brain injury in the amnesic patient N.A. based on magnetic resonance imaging. *Society for Neuroscience* **13**(2):1454, 1987.

Swanson LW, Kohler C: Anatomical evidence for direct projections from the entorhinal area to the entire cortical mantle in the rat. *The Journal of Neuroscience* **6**(10):3010–3023, 1986.

Tranel D, Damasio A: Knowledge without awareness: An autonomic index of facial recognition by prosopagnosics. *Science* **228**:1453–1454, 1985.

Tranel D, Damasio A: Covert recognition of "signal" stimuli after bilateral amygdala damage. *Society for Neuroscience* **12**(1):21, 1986.

Tranel D, Damasio A: Autonomic (covert) discrimination of familiar stimuli in patients with visual agnosia. *Neurology* **37**:129, and *Society for Neuroscience* **13**:1453, 1987.

Tranel D, Damasio A: Nonconscious face recognition in patients with face agnosia. *Behavioural Brain Research* **30**:235–249, 1988.

Tranel D, Damasio A, Damasio H: Impaired autonomic responses to emotional and social stimuli in patients with bilateral orbital damage and acquired sociopathy. *Society for Neuroscience*. Abstract, vol. 14, 1988.

Tranel D, Damasio A, Damasio H: Intact recognition of facial expression, gender, and age in patients with impaired recognition of face identity. *Neurology* **38**:680–696, 1988.

Tranel D, Biller J, Damasio H, Adams HP, Cornell S: Global aphasia without hemiparesis. *Archives of Neurology* **44**:304–308, 1987.

Triesman A, Gelade G. A feature-integration theory of attention. *Cognitive Neuropsychology* **12**:97–136, 1980.

Tulving E: Episodic and semantic memory. In Tulving E, Donaldson W (eds): *Organization of Memory*. New York, Academic Press, 1972.

Ungerleider LG, Mishkin M: Two cortical visual systems. In Ingle DJ, Mansfield RJW, Goodale MA (eds): *The Analysis of Visual Behavior*. Cambridge, MA, MIT Press, 1982.

Van Essen DC: Functional organization of primate visual cortex. In Peters A, Jones EG (eds): *Cerebral Cortex*, pp 259–329. New York, Plenum, 1985.

Van Essen D, Maunsell J. Hierarchical organization and functional streams in the visual cortex. *Trends in Neuroscience* **63**:370–375, 1983.

Van Hoesen GW: The primate parahippocampal gyrus: New insights regarding its cortical connections. *Trends in Neurosciences* **5**:345–350, 1982.

Van Hoesen, Damasio A: Neural correlates of the cognitive impairment in Alzheimer's disease. In Plum F (ed): Higher Functions of the Nervous System, pp 871–898. *The Handbook of Physiology*. American Physiological Society, Bethesda, MD, 1987.

Victor M, Adams R, Collins G: *The Wernicke-Korsakoff Syndrome*, ed 2. Philadelphia, F.A. Davis, 1988.

Vignolo LA, Boccardi E, Caverni L: Unexpected CT-scan findings in global aphasia. *Cortex* **22:**55–69, 1986.

Warrington EK, Shallice T: Category specific semantic impairments. *Brain* **107:**829–854, 1984.

Wernicke C: *Der aphasische Symptomencomplex*. Breslau, Cohn and Weigert, 1874.

Zeki SM: Colour coding in the superior temporal sulcus of rhesus monkey visual cortex. *Proceedings of the Royal Society of London* (Biol) **197:**195–223, 1977.

Zihl J, Von Cramon D, Mai N: Selective disturbance of movement vision after bilateral brain damage. *Brain* **106:**313–340, 1983.

3
COMPUTERIZED TOMOGRAPHY AND MAGNETIC RESONANCE STUDIES

Neuropathological Detection

The identification of neuropathological changes using computerized X-ray tomography depends on the detection, within a given brain region, of an X-ray absorption that departs from the standard normative value. In other words, given a certain type of brain tissue in a specified anatomical location, the presence of edema, infarction, or tumor will alter the standard X-ray absorption for that region and thus produce an abnormal image.

With magnetic resonance, the identification depends on the pathological brain region producing a locally different rate of hydrogen proton spinning after the brain is exposed to a magnetic field. In other words, after the brain is subjected to a magnetic field, with varied magnetic pulse sequence parameters, the presence of a pathological region due to edema, infarction, or tumor will determine hydrogen proton spinning rates within the area that are different from what normally would be expected for the given anatomical structure subjected to the same magnetic pulse sequence. Lesion detection sensitivity with either method varies according to the following factors: (a) the specific procedure, (b) the nature of the pathology, (c) the stage at which the imaging measurement is made in relation to the onset of the pathological process; and (d) the quality of the equipment and proficiency of the technique.

As with any detection procedure, the potential for false negatives or false positives is considerable, its magnitude depending, in any given instance, on the concerted weight of the factors previously

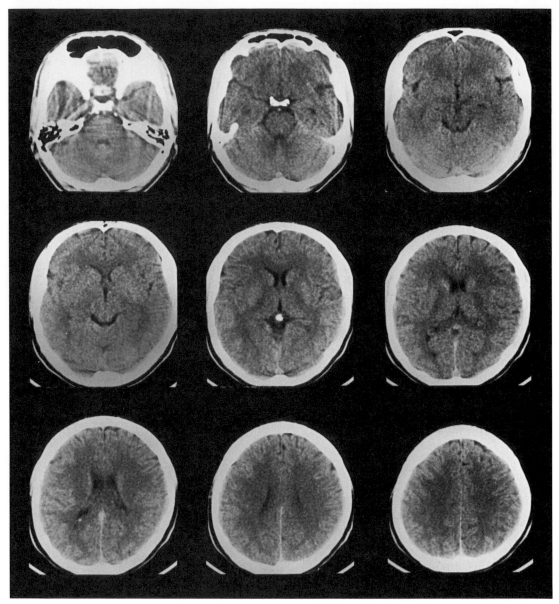

(A)

FIGURE 3.1. CT *without* contrast (A) obtained 10 days after a 28-year-old patient developed a severe aphasia due to a middle cerebral artery infarct. The images are entirely normal. Note the absence of any region of decreased density and the normal shape of cortical sulci, that is, the lack of effacement of cortical sulci.

CT of the same patient (B) obtained after intravenous injection of contrast material, 24 hours apart. Note the large area of increased density corresponding to Gray Matter Enhancement (GME) in the posterior frontal region, all of the insula, part of the anterior portion of the superior temporal gyrus, the transverse gyri of Heschl, the posterior portion of the superior temporal gyrus, the inferior portion of the supramarginal gyrus, and the head of the caudate and lenticular nucleus.

The patient had an unusual aphasia. The linguistic performance conformed to the category of Wernicke's aphasia, but the paucity of speech was atypical.

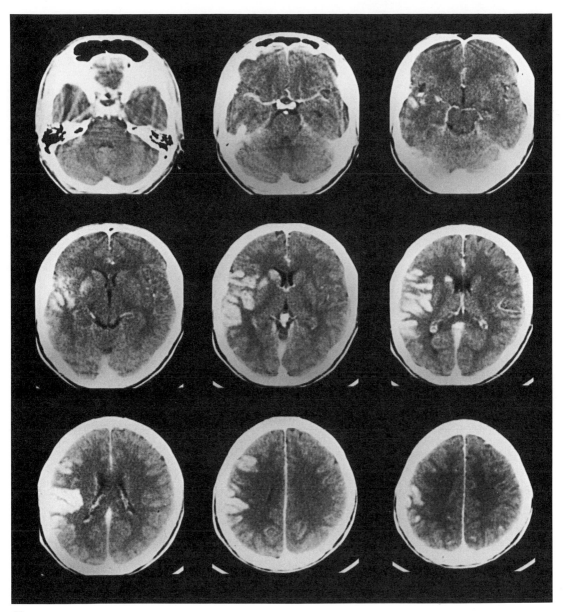

(B)

listed. For example, it is well accepted that CT is often negative in the first 24 hours after an infarct, but will become positive in the following days because the early pathological changes may fail to alter the X-ray absorption. However, this is not always true. Figure 3.1A shows the CT of a 28-year-old, right-handed man who suddenly developed a mild hemiparesis and aphasia. This plain CT, obtained without a contrast-enhancing injection, 10 days after the event, revealed no abnormality. At this time, the hemiparesis had

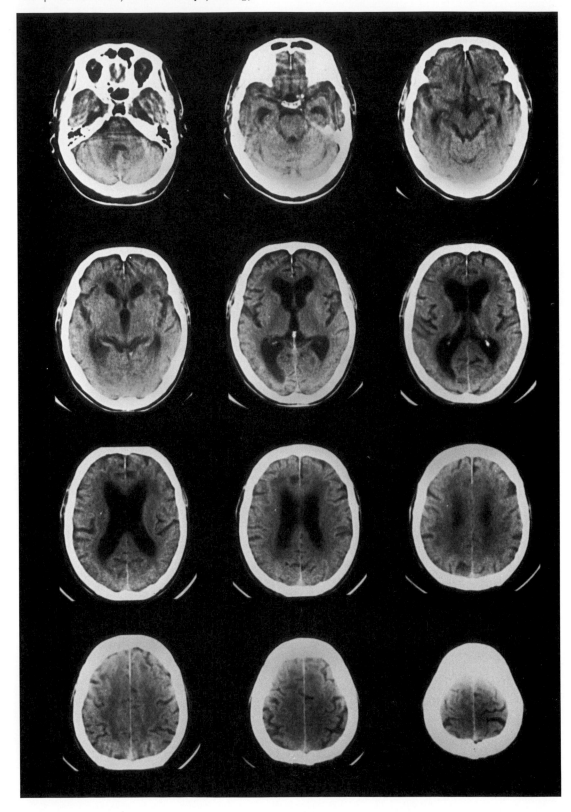

resolved but the language deficit, still present, was classified as a severe Wernicke's aphasia. This indicated that the patient had suffered a completed stroke and not just a transient ischemic attack (TIA). Is it that the stroke was so small that it was below the resolution of this late generation CT scanner? Why then was the CT "normal"? The problem in this case is that, at this particular epoch after stroke onset, the CT should be performed after the injection of a contrast-enhancing substance because changes in the infarcted tissue at this stage cause it to absorb X-rays at the same rate as normal tissue. The injection of a contrast substance increases the density of the infarcted region because contrast seeps out of damaged vessels in the region of the damage. As can be seen in Figure 3.1B, when contrast was added, the CT was indeed abnormal and showed a large area of increased density that corresponded to gray matter enhancement in the stroke region.

This also illustrates the fact that some so-called false negative instances may result from faulty use of the available techniques.

Even assuming state-of-the-art techniques, sensitive equipment working in the appropriate mode, and appropriate utilization of knowledge regarding the nature and timing of the pathological process, there are limits beyond which neuroimaging procedures cannot go. In most circumstances, it is impossible to guarantee the entire structural and functional intactness of neural tissue in the surround of focal lesions, even if it does appear intact by all available accounts. All that is permissible is an informed and well-reasoned guess whose probability of correctness will be higher or lower, depending on the observer's expertise and wisdom.

Neither CT nor MR are able to detect certain forms of cellular and subcellular pathology except indirectly. An example is degenerative dementia of either the Alzheimer or the Pick type, especially in the process's early phases. It is now clear that in Alzheimer's dementia the mesial temporal region is the primordial pathology site (Hyman et al, 1984, 1986), and yet, CT or MR images may be deceptively normal when neuropsychological assessment already reveals profound cerebral dysfunction. Dynamic neuroimaging using emission tomography procedures, of either the single-photon type (SPET), or positron type (PET), may show changes in cerebral blood flow or metabolism, while CT or MR continue to be structurally normal. An example can be seen in Figure 3.2. At the time CT was

---

FIGURE 3.2. CT of a 81-year-old man with a severe dementia involving varied aspects of cognition. The image is deceptively normal and does not even reveal "cortical" atrophy; that is, the cerebral sulci are not larger than normal. The only mild abnormality is the size of the ventricles. They are slightly enlarged, especially in the temporal horns (center cut in top row).

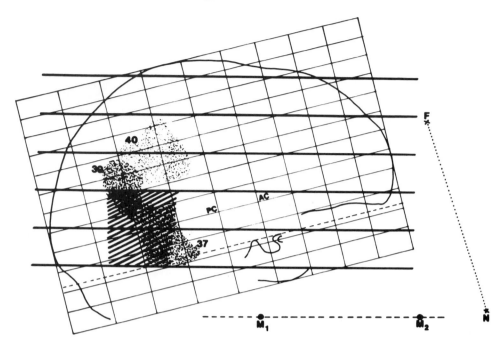

FIGURE 3.4. Talairach's *quadrilatere* construed around the lateral skull X-ray of the patient in Figure 3.3 (Talairach and Szikla, 1967). The X-ray was obtained at the time of the SPET study (see image of X-ray in Figure 3.5). Radioopaque markers were placed next to the external auditory canal (M_1) and the cantus of the eye (M_2). These two markers served to align the head so that the cuts obtained with the Tomomatic were parallel to the line passing through these two points. Two additional markers were placed on the nose (N) and forehead (F), at a distance of 10 cm from each other. These were used to calculate the magnification factor of the X-ray and permitted the marking of lines corresponding to the Tomomatic cuts, which were placed at a fixed distance from the baseline defined by M_1 and M_2. The areas of low radiosignal detected in the SPET scan were transposed to the lateral view of the skull (hatched area).

Talairach's *quadrilatere* allows the read-out of the involved region by plotting the stereotactic localization of the cortical surface of the brain (dotted regions identified by Brodmann's numbers). In this case, the low signal areas coincide with the posterior temporo-occipito-parietal junction, largely corresponding to area 37 of Brodmann's map.

Localization of areas of abnormal metabolism or blood flow seen in PET studies can be made in a similar way (see Fox et al, 1985).

obtained, this 81-year-old patient showed severe impairment in virtually all aspects of cognitive function. His CT, however, is unremarkable. On the other hand, a contemporaneous SPET scan [Figure 3.3] shows marked decrease of radiosignal in both posterior temporal regions [see Figures 3.4 and 3.5 for the localization method used with SPET]. At autopsy, some years later, the typical pathological changes of Alzheimer's disease confirmed the diagnosis.

Decreased radiosignal in posterior temporal and temporo-parietal regions appears to be quite characteristic of Alzheimer's dementia (Chase et al, 1984; Foster et al, 1984; Friedland et al, 1983; Rezai et al., 1985). (This is probably the consequence of *both* local patho-

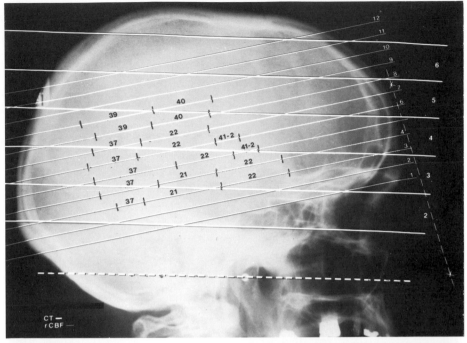

(A)

(B)

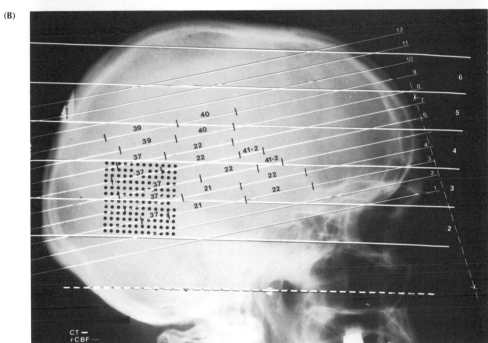

FIGURE 3.5. Photographs of the same skull X-ray used for the construction in Figure 3.4 with the line markings corresponding to the SPET study (thick lines). The lines corresponding to the CT cuts, as seen on the pilot scan of the CT, were transposed onto the same image (thin lines). The boundaries of the different gyri of the temporal and parietal lobe seen on CT were marked on these lines and are identified by the numbers of Brodmann's cytoarchitectonic areas (A). In (B), the area of low signal seen in SPET is also plotted on this image (dotted area), permitting the direct reading of the involved region.

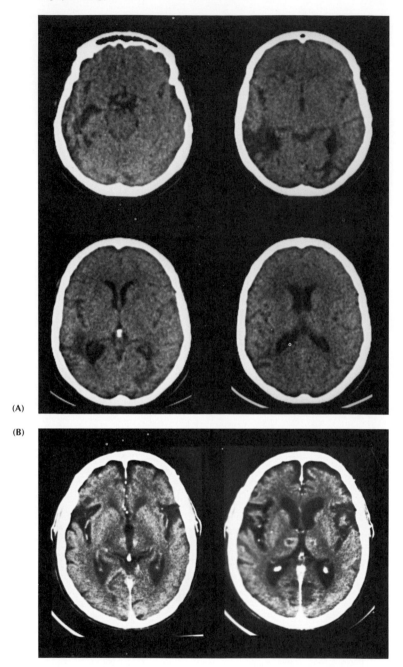

(A)

(B)

FIGURE 3.7. CT (A) of the patient in Figure 3.6A. Note the bilateral areas of decreased density in the temporo-occipital region. (MR of this patient can be seen in Figure 2.8).

CT (B) of the patient in Figure 3.6B. Note the bilateral mesial thalamic infarcts.

logical changes and local physiological changes brought about by anterior temporal lesions; see A. Damasio, to be published). However, we have to caution against overreliance on such images for an Alzheimer's disease diagnosis. These dynamic changes are not pathognomonic of the disease. Patients with cerebrovascular accidents occurring bilaterally in the posterior cerebral circulation territory may have similar patterns in SPET [Figure 3.6A and B]. In such cases, however, the SPET images are due to symmetrical structural damage in the occipitotemporal regions, as in case A, or in the thalamus, as in case B [see Figure 3.7]. As a result of bilateral occipitotemporal infarctions, the patient in Figures 3.6A and 3.7A had prosopagnosia, and the patient in Figures 3.6B and 3.7B developed disturbances in alertness and attention. However, neither had any deficits suggesting degenerative dementia.

In moderate to advanced stages of Alzheimer's disease, CT and MR may show marked and fairly widespread cerebral atrophy or ventricular enlargement. Such an example can be found in Figure 3.8. This type of finding led us and other researchers to attempt a quantification of the ventricular size changes in dementia patients. The aim was to obtain an indirect quantitative anatomical index for use in the evaluation of such patients because the likely focal sites of damage remained so structurally normal (H. Damasio et al, 1983). We found that when the comparison was made to truly normal individuals of the same age (subjects without any neurological disorder or any other condition that might influence normal, nervous system function), we were able to detect the scans of demented patients with a 77% accuracy rate.

In Pick's disease, autopsy studies have shown repeatedly that the characteristic pathology is especially evident in the frontal and anterior temporal cortices (Escourolle & Poirier, 1978). In some cases, anatomical analysis of CT or MR of patients with progressive dementia does reveal severe localized atrophy in those regions, as can be demonstrated in Figures 3.9 and 3.10. In other cases, the slow progress of cognitive decline noted with sequential neuropsychological investigations can be matched by specific anatomical changes, as seen in the example shown in Figure 3.11 (see also Graff-Radford et al, to be published).

In brief, the value of lesion studies in degenerative dementias based on the currently available *in-vivo* imaging technology remains limited.

The Choice of Neuropathological Specimens

As noted previously, the choice of pathological specimen is a major methodological consideration. The neuropathological characteristics of an infarction, an intraparenchymal hemorrhage, or different types

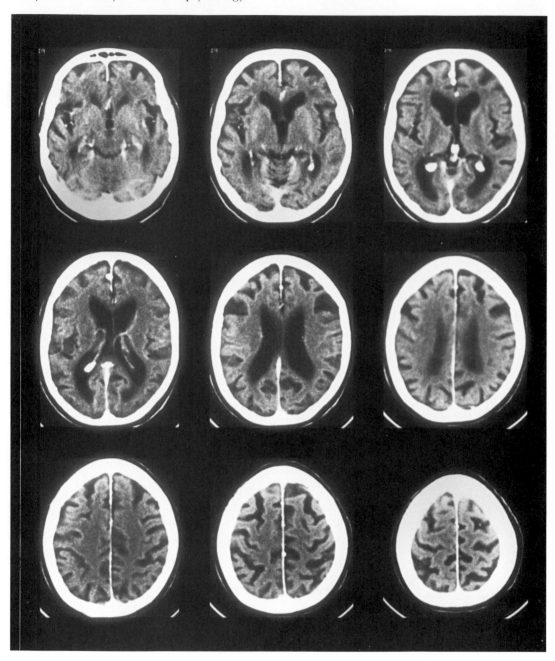

FIGURE 3.8. CT of a 67-year-old woman with severe dementia. At the time of this scan, the condition had progressed slowly for five years. Compare this with the CT of Figure 3.2. Note that in this case, the ventricles are unequivocally enlarged and that there is widespread cortical atrophy (sulcal enlargement).

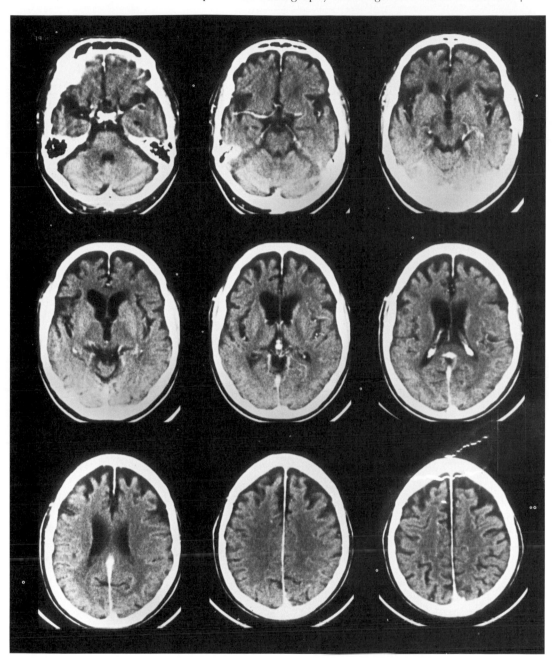

FIGURE 3.9. CT of a 72-year-old man with progressive memory loss over several years. Note that there is marked atrophy in the frontal lobes from the lowest cut onward. Atrophy also exists in the anterior temporal lobes, most notably in the first three cuts. The posterior temporal region and the parietal and occipital lobes are all remarkably normal; that is, the sulci are not enlarged.

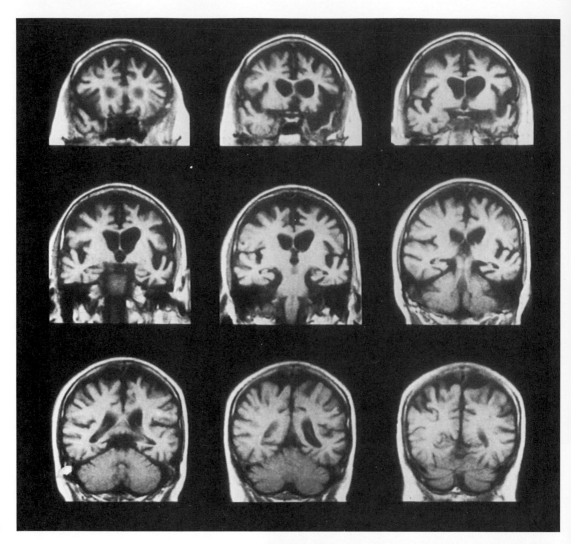

(A)

FIGURE 3.10. MR of the patient in Figure 3.9 obtained three years later. Coronal T_1 weighted images can be seen on top (A). In (B), there is a midsagittal cut used as a pilot for the coronal cuts.

The frontal lobe atrophy is easily observable in the sagittal cut. It stops sharply at the boundary with the primary motor region in the posterior sector of the frontal cortices.

Note that the patient's head is hyperextended and, for this reason, the cuts are in a different angle from the usual coronal cuts. The angle is here indicated by the dotted line (B). This is why casual inspection of the coronal cuts might suggest that the atrophy extends into the parietal and possibly occipital regions, when, in fact, it is strictly limited to the frontal lobe. Note that the frontal lobe is still seen in the upper portion of the last cut, a cut that due to its peculiar angulation passes through the posterior edge of the cerebellum.

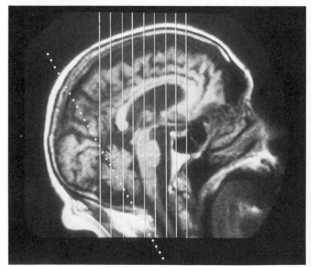

(B)

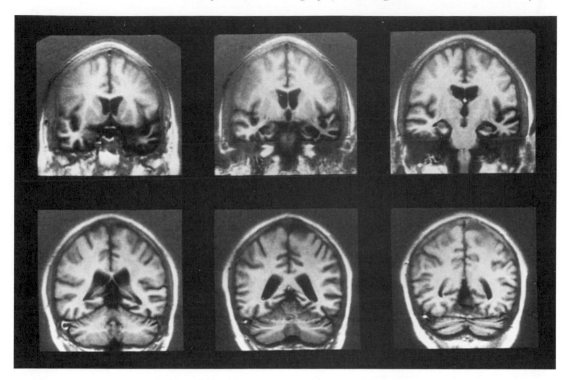

FIGURE 3.11. MR (T₁ weighted images) of a 59-year-old man who gradually developed a difficulty in retrieving the names of specific people, places, and objects. His retrieval of nonspecific names—the names of properties or functions of objects, for instance—remained intact, as did all aspects of nonverbal memory. Other than the lexical retrieval disturbance, the patient's language remained intact, and so did his intelligence, measured by IQ and judged by his continued ability to run his business interests soundly. Note the remarkable atrophy of the left temporal region. The entire temporal lobe is affected, but the atrophy is particularly impressive in the anterior, mesial, and inferior sectors. The anterior mesial aspect (fifth or parahippocampal gyrus, fourth and third gyri) is virtually gone. The first and second temporal gyri can be traced but are thinned out. It is only at a level posterior to the transverse gyri of Heschl (seen in cut 3) that the structures appear normal again. In the first two cuts, the right temporal lobe also shows some signs of atrophy, but far less than the left. All other brain structures appear normal.

Post-mortem microscopic studies confirmed that the neuropathological process was largely circumscribed to the atrophied sector, as a result of Pick's disease.

of tumors are entirely different. For this reason, their neuropsychological manifestations can be expected to be quite different, even with apparently similar lesion loci.

Nonhemorrhagic Infarction

Nonhemorrhagic infarctions provide the best specimens for neuroanatomical investigation and correlation with neuropsychological findings. Cerebral infarctions entail actual destruction of brain parenchyma. The infarcted area is eventually replaced by scar tissue

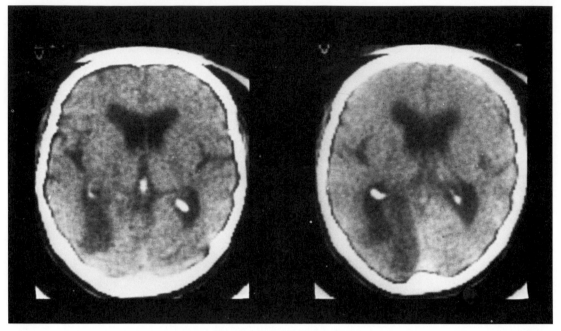

(A)

FIGURE 3.12. CT (A) of a 68-year-old man who developed alexia without agraphia. He was unable to read sentences and most single words; even single letters posed difficulties. Writing to dictation or spontaneously was intact, as was Spelling. Note the characteristic location of the lesion involving the left mesial occipital cortices (areas 17, and inferior 18, 19 mesially), the occipitotemporal tran-sition (the region striding the fifth occipital and fifth temporal, or parahippocampal gyri). The lesion extends into the paraventricular region. The *paraventricular region* is the zone located beside, beneath, behind, and immediately above the occipital horn. We have determined that damage in this area is virtually necessary for pure alexia to appear (Damasio & Damasio, 1983).

and by cerebrospinal fluid. CT or MR in the chronic state provide a clear demarcation of the infarct. In CT, the damage is depicted as an area of decreased density, which appears as a darker area in terms of the gray scales used in the images. In MR, it becomes a dark area in T_1 weighted images, and a white bright signal region in T_2 weighted images. In the chronic state, the images map with great precision the actual area of macroscopic brain destruction.

Even older-generation CT scanners permitted a remarkable mapping of infarction, as can be judged from the comparison of CT images and the result of occasional autopsies. Figure 3.12 provides an example of the quality that has been available for quite some time. It shows the CT of a patient with pure alexia and a right homonymous hemianopia caused by a left mesial occipital infarct. On the CT [Figure 3.12A], an area of normal-appearing brain tissue can be seen, surrounded by images of infarction. The corre-

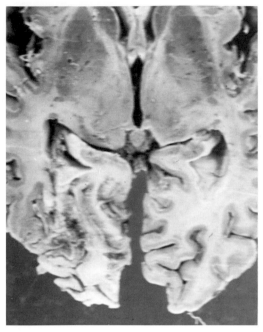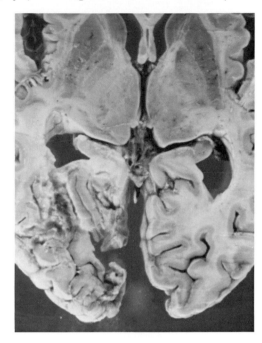

(B)

Note that in cut 2 an area of normal-looking brain density occurs between the two low-density regions.

Brain cuts (B) obtained at autopsy in the same plane as the CT. Note the preserved gyrus in cut 2, corresponding precisely to the normal density area detected by CT. (Modified from Damasio & Damasio, *Neurology* 33:1573–1583, 1983). In re-

cent years there has been amazing progress in the conceptualization of the reading process from the cognitive viewpoint. But the link between those new ideas and the anatomical data described above remains to be made.

sponding cut obtained at autopsy [Figure 3.12B] indicates the correctness of the image, as it reveals an area in which a fold of cortex has been spared, almost as an island surrounded by entirely destroyed brain parenchyma. (See also the example in Figure 2.9).

Herpes Encephalitis

A comparably reliable anatomical detail of damaged brain structure exists in only one other neuropathological type: herpes simplex encephalitis. This is because the virus has a particular affinity for only a limited set of brain structures, mostly within the limbic system, and because it destroys those areas rather completely, by a mechanism that includes vascular collapse. Both CT and MR produce extremely accurate images of the involved areas [see Figures 3.13 and 3.14, and also 2.13].

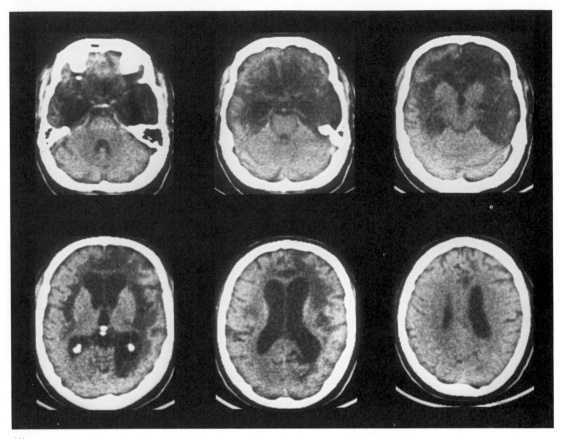

(A)

FIGURE 3.13. CT (A) and corresponding templates (B) of the patient in Figure 2.11 who had herpes simplex encephalitis. This CT was obtained seven years after the illness. The presence of brain damage is unequivocal. It involves both hemispheres in the mesial temporal region (hippocampal gyrus, amygdala), as well as the fourth and third temporal gyri, the temporal poles, and the basal

Other Pathological Specimens

In practically all other varieties of neuropathological insult, the precise anatomical definition of lesions is more problematic, and so is the functional impact of the lesion itself. For instance, earlier in the course gliomas infiltrate brain tissue by dislocating local populations of neurons but often do not destroy them. It is for this reason that they may grow for long periods of time without overt clinical manifestations. The region of low or high density seen on the CT of such tumors corresponds not only to the tumor tissue itself but also to surrounding edema and even to functionally competent brain tissue. Even when we look at a region where an abnormal signal definitely exists, this does not mean necessarily that the brain parenchyma is destroyed, or that the area is functionally inoperative. Nor

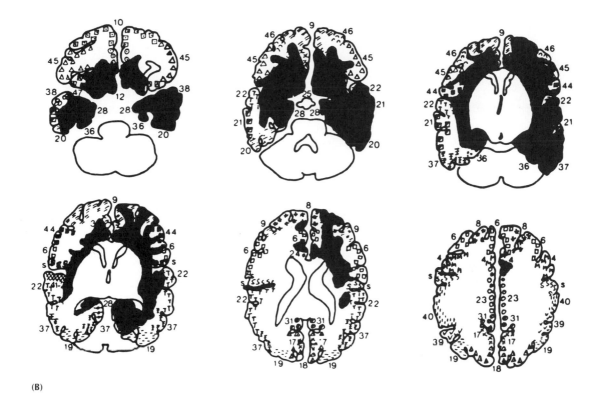

(B)

forebrain region. The right hemisphere is even more involved, both in lateral portions of the temporal lobe and in the occipitotemporal junction and the frontal lobe. Chronic CT can detect this kind of damage and permit a good anatomical analysis, although the amount of anatomical detail provided by MR is far superior (see Figure 2.13).

can we be sure that an area without apparent abnormality is free of tumor. Because of this, we do not believe that patients with tumors are a material of choice for brain/behavior studies, although clearly there are notable exceptions.

Figures 3.15 and 3.16 show the MR of a young patient referred to our service after a generalized seizure. The "blind" and "unbiased" interpretation of these images would lead us to think that this is the image of a cerebrovascular accident involving temporal and parietal branches of the left middle cerebral artery. The damaged area corresponds to posterior language-related regions in the temporal and parietal lobes. If a prediction of the behavioral presentation of the patient were made on such an anatomical basis, we would expect a fluent aphasia of the Wernicke type, provided the patient was left-hemisphere dominant for language (which would be

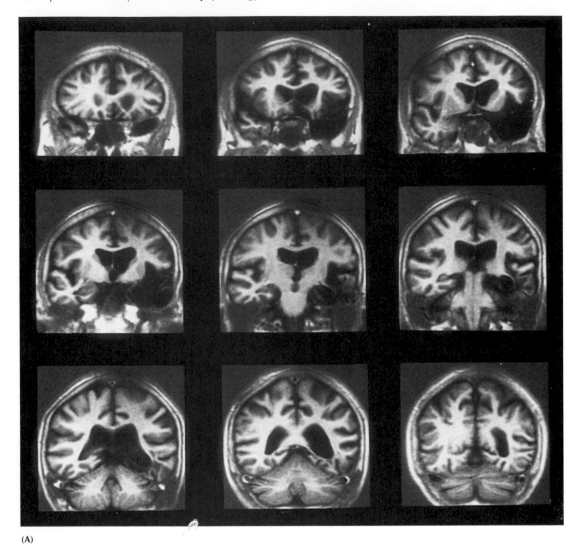

(A)

FIGURE 3.14. T$_1$ weighted MR (A) and corresponding templates (B) of a 62-year-old, right-handed woman who had herpes simplex encephalitis. The sequela was a circumscribed verbal memory defect. She has difficulty retrieving old specific names and learning new specific names. Her recall and recognition for nonverbal material and her nonverbal learning are intact.

The MR shows that the area of abnormally low signal is limited to the left hemisphere and involves the pole of the temporal lobe extending into all of the mesial temporal region (amygdala, hip-

reasonable, given her full right-handedness and the absence of left-handers in immediate relatives). The patient, however, had entirely normal language and speech. The problem was that these images were not caused by a vascular lesion but rather by the presence of a glioma, later confirmed with a biopsy. The example demonstrates that the currently available neuroimaging techniques do not allow a "blind" reading of abnormal patterns. They cannot diagnose micro-

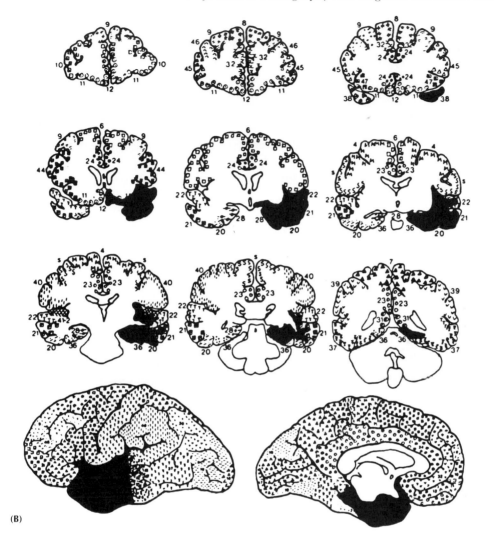

(B)

pocampal and fourth temporal gyri, as well as inferior, medial, and superior temporal gyri up to the level of the primary auditory cortices). The posterior portion of the superior, medial, and inferior temporal gyri is intact (this includes posterior area 22, or Wernicke's area, and area 37). The anterior insula is destroyed, as is the basal forebrain region. Our evidence indicates that structures in the left anterior temporal region are critical for the learning and retrieval of reference lexical entries such as nouns and verbs.

scopic pathology reliably. Nor can they reliably guarantee, except in instances of stroke and some forms of encephalitis, that an abnormal signal means dead brain tissue or even inoperant brain structure. The latter point was made by Anderson, Damasio, and Tranel (1988) when they compared the neuropsychological profile of patients with confirmed gliomas to that of patients with strokes in the same regions. Invariably, the stroke cases, even with lesions that were

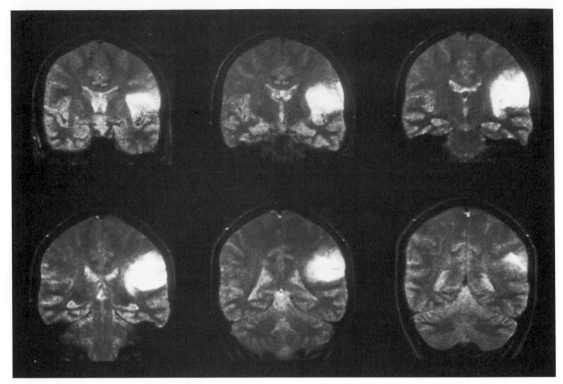

(A)

FIGURE 3.15. T$_2$ weighted MR (A) and corresponding templates (B) of a 28-year-old, right-handed
woman who suddenly developed generalized seizures. She had no focal neurological defect, and
language and speech were normal. The area of
abnormally bright signal in the left hemisphere involves most of the superior temporal gyrus (including the transverse gyri of Heschl, or Brodmann's areas 41 and 42, and area 22 immediately
behind, or Wernicke's area). The abnormal signal
also occupies most of the supramarginal gyrus (area
40) and borders the anterior portion of the angular gyrus (area 39). In the rostral direction, it reaches
the postcentral gyrus (with areas 3, 1, 2, or pri-

more limited, had more severe neuropsychological deficits than the
tumor cases. Compare the case in Figures 3.15 and 3.16 with the
patient in Figure 3.17, who had severe fluent aphasia due to a stroke.

Naturally, those results do not mean that tumors cause no measurable deficits, but rather that the magnitude of disturbance is generally small, at least in the early stages.

Surgical Ablations

An exceptional instance in which tumor cases are acceptable is that
of subjects in whom meningiomas have been excised and a circumscribed ablation of brain tissue has been performed during surgery.
Provided these patients are stable, the just mentioned cases are entirely appropriate to establish a link between the anatomical site of

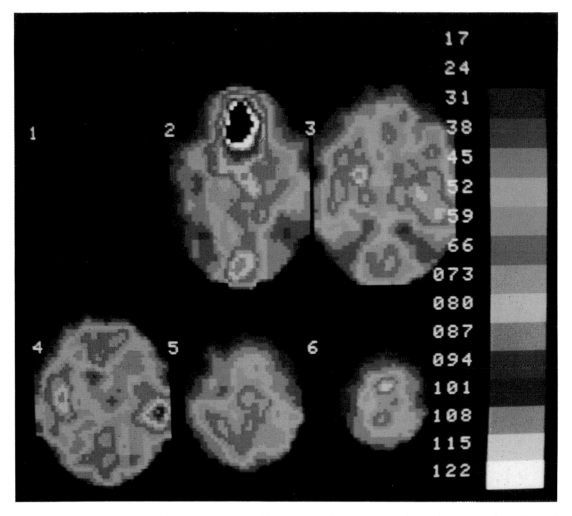

FIGURE 3.3. SPET obtained at rest with the To-momatic 64 (Medimatic, Denmark). The patient is the same one studied in Figure 3.2. Note that the two posterior temporal regions show a very low radiosignal level. Otherwise, the levels and distribution of radiosignal are normal. The left hemisphere is on the left and the right hemisphere on the right. The scale on the right-hand side indicates the correspondence between the value of regional cerebral blood flow and the color code. Note that the region of the visual cortices (posterior midline zone in the first two cuts) shows high values of radiosignal. This is because the patients are studied in a resting position with eyes *open* in a regularly lit room.

FIGURE 3.6. SPET (A) obtained at rest in a 67-year-old woman who developed severe prosopagnosia after bilateral occipitotemporal infarcts. Note that the areas of low radiosignal seen in this situation are placed in the same areas of low radiosignal seen in cases of Alzheimer's disease (see Figure 3.3).

Similarly placed low radiosignal areas (B) in the case of an 81-year-old man with bilateral thalamic infarcts. At onset, he presented with severe lethargy, and was virtually unarousable. After somnolence cleared, testing revealed a disturbance of attention, defective memory, and emotional bluntness. Six months later, he was well-oriented and had only mild memory defects. SPET was obtained in the chronic stage.

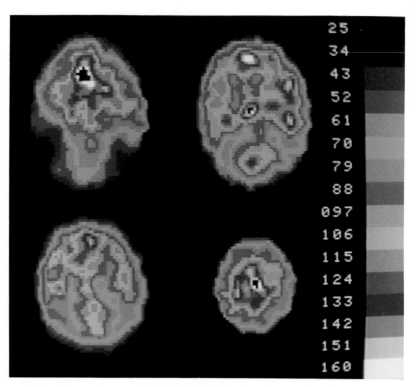

(A)

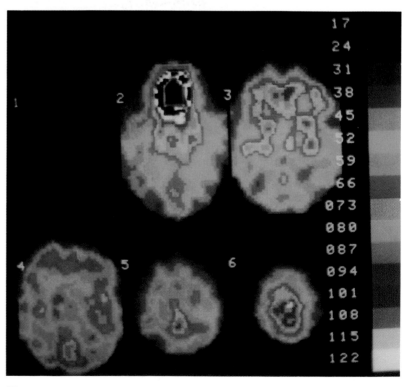

(B)

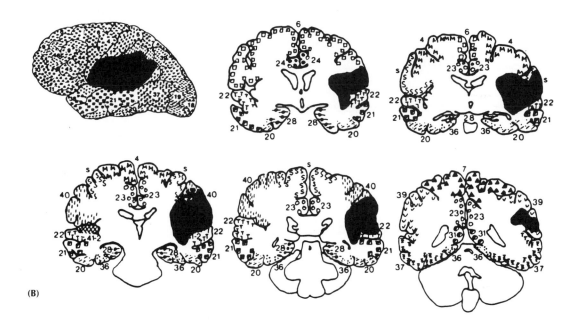

(B)

mary sensory cortices). The insula and the temporal isthmus are entirely covered by the area of abnormal signal. The lateral diagram of the left hemisphere shows the lateral and external projection of the extent of the abnormality.

If dysfunction in these areas had been due to an infarction, it would certainly have caused a major aphasia. Yet, this patient had normal language and only a minimal speech impediment, best described as an occasional stutter. This is because the lesion was due to a glioma. Biopsy revealed it to be an astrocytoma Grade V. (Compare with the case in Figure 3.17).

the ablation and the neuropsychological profile obtained *after* the ablation took place. An example of this use can be found in the study by Eslinger and Damasio (1985) of a patient who had had a restricted frontal lobe resection to treat an orbital meningioma and had developed severe social conduct disturbances as a consequence of the resection. The anatomical investigation, conducted eight years after the resection, showed damage in orbital and lower mesial frontal cortices and revealed only negligible damage to dorsolateral cortices and higher mesial cortices. In particular, the left dorsolateral cortices and their underlying white matter was intact. Coronal images also allowed us to establish that the basal forebrain region remained intact [Figure 2.11].

Patients who have had ablations for seizure treatment also afford a good opportunity for behavioral and anatomical studies. In those

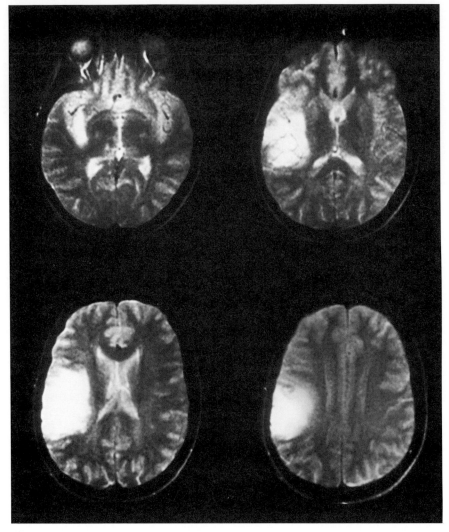

(A)

FIGURE 3.16. T$_2$ weighted MR (A) and corresponding templates (B) of the patient discussed in Figure 3.15. Here, the transverse cuts are depicted together with the correspondiing templates. As expected, the areas of damage are the same as in Figure 3.15. Compare this case with the example in Figure 3.17.

cases, MR obtained with T$_1$ weighted images can help delineate the extent of brain tissue removal with extraordinary precision [Figure 3.18], although some caution is recommended in the interpretation of the material. Patients who undergo surgical removals of brain tissue for the treatment of uncontrollable seizures may have developmental brain defects and are likely to have had some degree of abnormal brain organization before surgery, not to mention cerebral changes consequent to long-standing seizural discharges. The

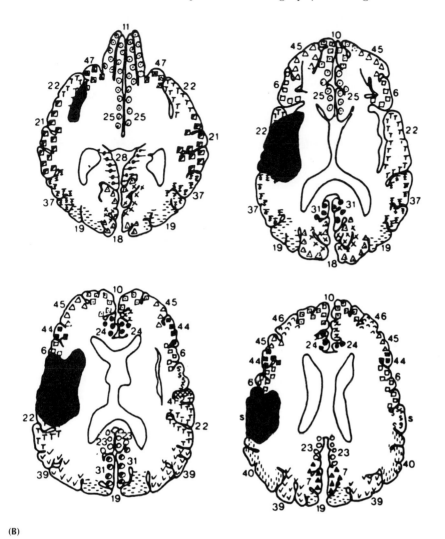

(B)

images of a 14-year-old patient who underwent a left temporal lobectomy to control partial complex seizures is a case in point. Before surgery, imaging studies had revealed an arachnoid cyst in the
anterior tip of the temporal lobe. Figures 3.19 and 3.20 demonstrate the extent of the temporal lobe removal as seen in the MR
images. The hippocampus and the overlying entorhinal cortex clearly
remained intact, possibly because the cyst may have "pushed" these
structures; that is, a resection with precisely the same rostro-caudal
extent in a normal individual would probably have encompassed the
hippocampal complex. After surgery, this patient had no detectable
neuropsychological deficits, namely no memory disturbance for verbal material, something that may be attributed to the intactness of
the left hippocampus. It is important to note that a superficial ob-

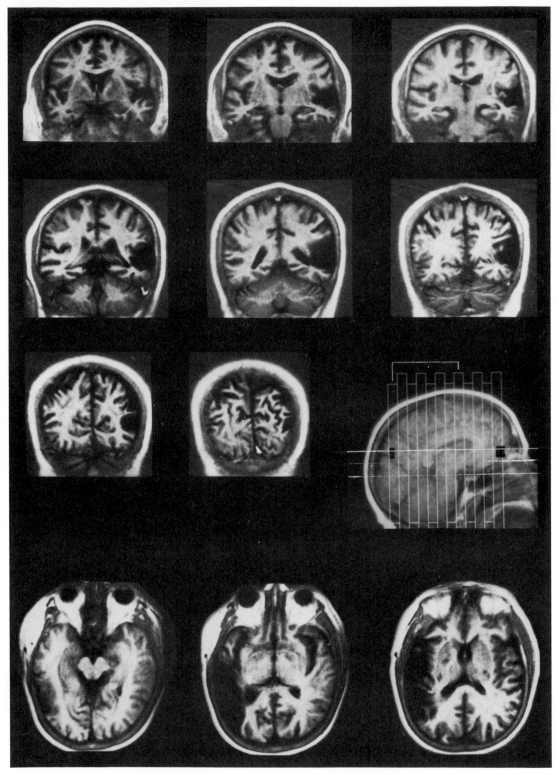

(A)

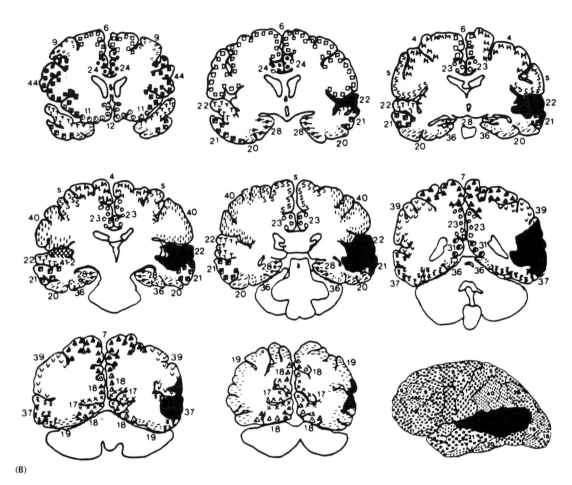

(B)

FIGURE 3.17. MR (A) and corresponding templates (B) of a 63-year-old, right-handed woman who suddenly developed a fluent aphasia. Acutely, her speech was marred by neologisms, but was well-articulated and had appropriate prosody. All aspects of formal language assessment were severely defective (this included aural comprehension of words and sentences; Token Test; visual, tactile, and auditory naming; sentence repetition; writing and reading). Even comprehension of a simple conversation was severely impaired.

Five months post-onset, at the time the MR was obtained, she was still severely aphasic. She presented then with "hyperfluent," pressured speech, and made numerous phonemic and semantic paraphasias. Her aural comprehension in conversation had improved somewhat, but was still defective. Formal language assessment still showed severe linguistic impairments.

The clinical profile conforms to the category of Wernicke's aphasia. As with other clinical categories, the label encompasses a highly heterogeneous group of aphasias, with different degrees of severity and varied outcomes. Lesion placement, education, intelligence, and neural language endowment are obvious factors behind the heterogeneity.

The T_1 weighted MR shows an area of low signal in the left temporal lobe that involves most of the superior temporal gyrus (only the most anterior portion is spared), including primary auditory cortices and Wernicke's area. The lesion extends into the middle temporal gyrus, mainly in its medial and posterior regions (areas 21 and 37), and the posterior portion of the insula, and goes slightly into the angular gyrus. (See also Figure 3.23A).

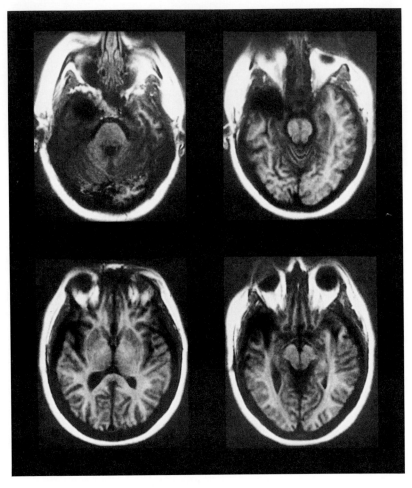

(A)

FIGURE 3.18. MR of a 32-year-old woman who underwent a left temporal lobectomy for the control of refractory seizures. The images are T_1 weighted and shown in transverse (A), coronal (B), and parasagittal (C), cuts. Although all images reveal the missing sector of the temporal lobe, the coronal cuts reveal it the best. Because of the fine resolution, several anatomical features can be clearly identified and allow a direct reading of the lesion. The entire pole of the temporal lobe is missing, as well as the anterior portion of the mesial temporal region (it includes the amygdala, the very anterior hypocampal formation, and the para-hippocampal gyrus; and the anterior-most portion of the fourth, third, and second temporal gyri). The first temporal gyrus is largely spared.

The resection practised in this patient was quite anterior and limited (the patient was fully right-handed and had language dominance in the left hemisphere, judging from her Wada Test). Seizure control improved remarkably. Although the patient did not develop an aphasia, she did note a decrease in her verbal learning (manifested, for instance, in the fact that she no longer can take telephone messages and communicate them accurately, unless she writes them down *pari passu*).

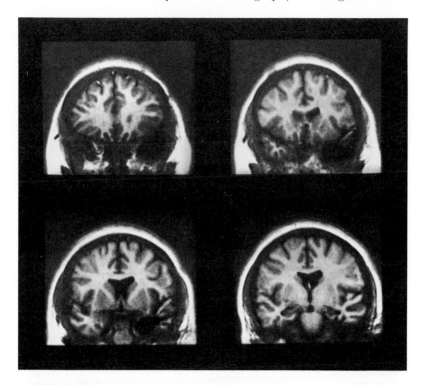

(B)

(C)

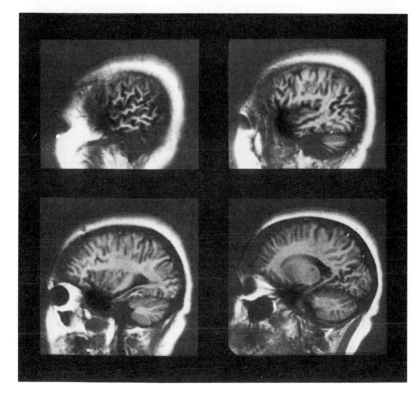

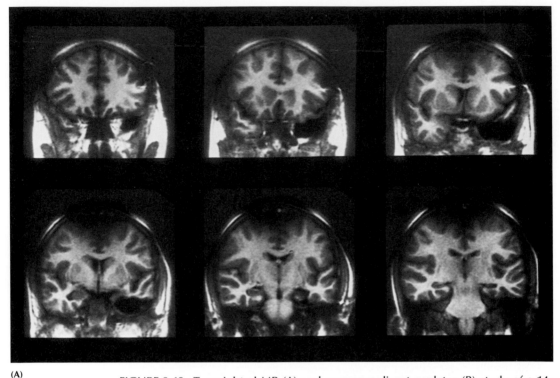

(A)

FIGURE 3.19. T$_1$ weighted MR (A) and corresponding templates (B) study of a 14-year-old boy who underwent a left temporal lobectomy for the treatment of uncontrollable partial complex seizures. The extent of the resection is readily visiible on the coronal cuts. It is important to note that the left hippocampus and parahippocampal gyrus are clearly identifiable, and that the resection is restricted to the anterior-most temporal lobe structures. The sparing of verbal learning abilities may well be explained by the preservation of the left hippocampal region.

servation of the scans might have led to the false impression that the hippocampal complex had been removed. If that were true, the normalcy of verbal learning would have to be explained by postulating that the entire left hippocampal complex would have been dysfunctional all along, given its paroxystic disruption by seizures and possible developmental abnormalities, and that even after its resection had been accomplished, little or no defect might have ensued because its function would have been assumed by the right hippocampus all along. In short, interpretation of brain/behavior correlations in such cases must be cautious.

Metastatic Lesions and Hemorrhagic Infarctions

One other exception should be mentioned in relation to isolated, well-defined, noninfiltrating metastatic lesions. When a patient has a single brain metastasis removed surgically and is studied in the stable, post-operative state, concomitantly with a good-quality CT or

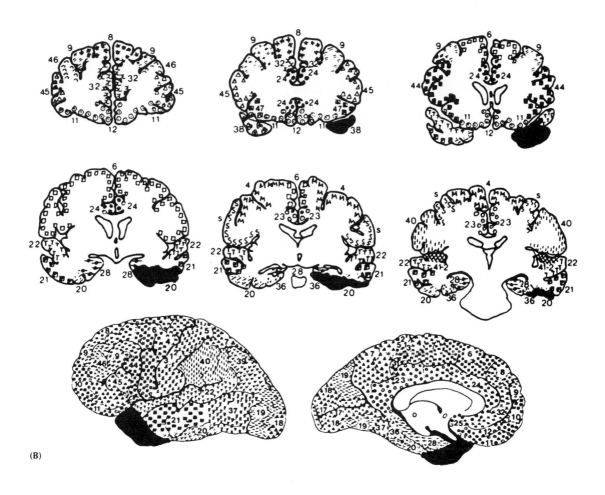

(B)

MR [see example in Figure 3.21], there is no reason why a correlate should not be established between neuropsychological deficits and anatomical site of lesion (Anderson et al, to be published).

Intracerebral hemorrhages behave in a mixed fashion, both by destroying neural tissue, as nonhemorrhagic infarctions do, and by producing a space-occupying blood collection that displaces neurons, as tumors do. During the acute phase of a hemorrhage, neither CT nor MR provides an accurate picture of the abnormality, because within the area of abnormal signal some neurons are truly destroyed, whereas others are simply displaced. Figure 3.22 shows two CT studies obtained in the acute phase of intracerebral hemorrhages, one involving the left hemisphere and the other, the right. At the time these CTs were performed, the two lesions shared many features. However, by the time the chronic MRs of these same two patients were obtained, the anatomical outcomes were remarkably different [Figure 3.23].

In the chronic state, patient A was left with a large zone of de-

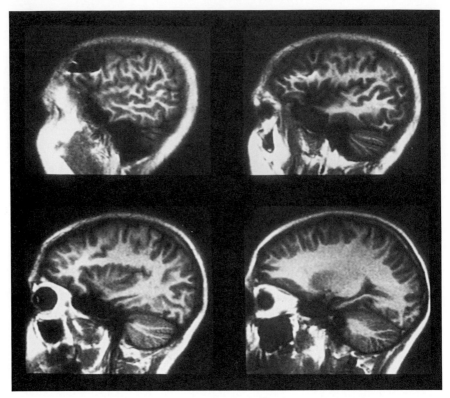

(A)

FIGURE 3.20. Parasagittal cuts (A) of the MR in Figure 3.19. The missing temporal lobe can be clearly traced. Note, however, that the hippocampus is clearly visible and undamaged in the last cut.

Transverse cuts (B) of same patient. Cut number 3 shows that the left entorhinal cortex is intact. Most of the superior temporal gyrus, the entorhinal region, and most of the hippocampus are intact. This may explain the absence of defects in verbal learning and retrieval.

struction in the posterior aspect of the temporal lobe (in areas 37 and 22), whereas patient B showed a slit-like defect undercutting most of the superior temporal gyrus and part of the supramarginal gyrus. The cortex itself sustained no damage. These cases demonstrate that it is only after the resolution of a hematoma that one may actually estimate the amount and location of tissue destruction. Only at that time can a good relation be established between the neuropsychological defect and the affected brain tissue.

In brief, when the purpose is to establish correlates between dysfunction and site of brain destruction, the specimens of choice are nonhemorrhagic infarction and herpes encephalitis. Surgical ablations performed for the treatment of meningiomas provide excellent experimental material. With few exceptions, other tumor material is not acceptable.

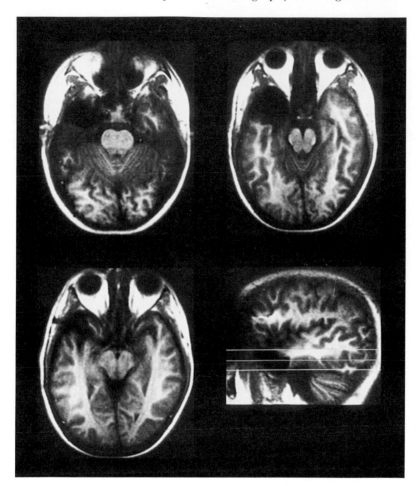

(B)

Timing CT and MR Data Collection

The timing of CT and MR data collection is of the essence, especially in relation to subjects with cerebrovascular disease, by far the most frequent and appropriate type of subject. Both CT and MR may fail to show *any* abnormality when obtained immediately after the occurrence of a stroke. With fourth-generation CT scanners, most images will be positive after 24 hours. This is certainly not the case in older scanners, however. Many CT studies obtained less than 24 hours after the onset of a stroke are negative. It is important to keep this in mind, especially when a patient with an acute stroke happens to have a CT that shows a well-demarcated area of low density with sharp margins. Such an image is normally not the image of an acute infarct and most certainly corresponds to a previous

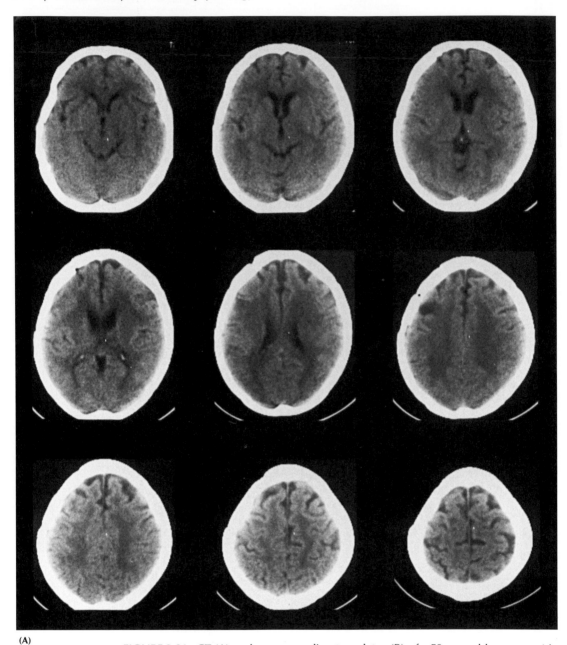

(A)

FIGURE 3.21. CT (A) and corresponding templates (B) of a 58-year-old woman with a single metastasis from lung carcinoma. This CT was obtained after surgical removal of the metastasis and stabilization of the patient's condition. The size of brain excision can be seen as a clearly demarcated area of low density in the left frontal lobe, in the pre-motor region, above the frontal operculum and just behind area 8 (see Anderson, A. Damasio and H. Damasio, to be published).

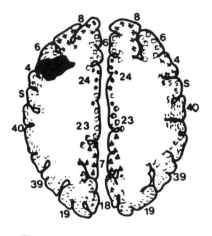

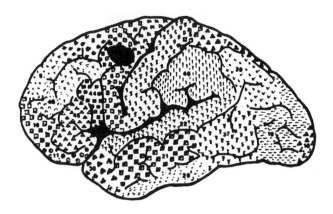

(B)

stroke that may even be unknown to the patient [see Figures 3.24 and 3.25].

Positive CT images obtained in the first week post-onset usually show areas of abnormality that are far larger than the region of actual structural damage because of confounding phenomena, for example, edema. This commonly occurs and means that the results of observations and experiments conducted at later epochs should not be correlated with the anatomical analysis performed on the acute images.

Figure 3.26 shows the MR of a patient with sudden fluent aphasia and alexia four days after the stroke. The abnormal signal area involves the middle temporal and most of the inferior temporal gyri extending all the way to the occipital lobe, posteriorly, and quite deeply into the white matter. The chronic scan of the same patient shows a more restricted area of damage [Figure 3.27]. This "shrinking" lesion phenomenon is observed with both MR and with CT.

When CT is obtained in the second or third week after a storke's onset, without IV infusion of a contrast-enhancing substance, the images are negative in a good number of cases [Figure 3.1A]. The image can change [as seen in Figure 3.28], even after a previous CT obtained immediately after the onset of the neurological symptoms showed a large area of decreased density [Figure 2.12]. On the other hand, in contrast-enchanced CT images, otherwise silent areas of infarction appear as areas of increased density (primarily due to seepage of contrast substance through the walls of newly formed vessels in the affected region; see Figures 3.1B and Figure 3.28B).

In the chronic stage, which we define as three months post-onset and beyond, most CT studies of infarction are unequivocally positive. Even then, however, when strokes are small and located close

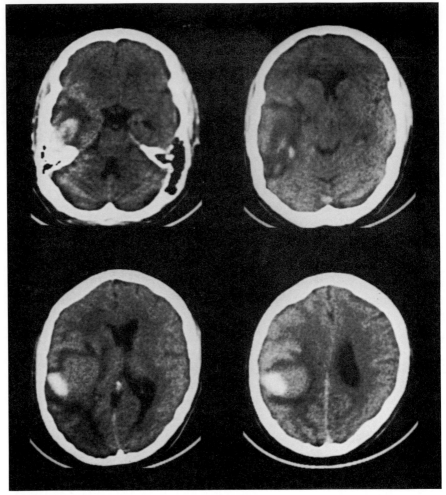

(A)

FIGURE 3.22. CTs of two cases of intracerebral hematoma, one in the left hemi-sphere (A) and one in the right (B). Both were obtained 10 days after the hemor-rhage occurred. At this stage, the images are remarkably similar. A large collection of blood, surrounded by a vast area of edema, is seen in the temporal lobe. There is shift of the midline structures. The images should be compared with those ob-tained in the chronic stage, after the hematomas were reabsorbed.

to a major sulcus or to the wall of a ventricle, the chronic CT may mislead the observer, resembling images of focal "atrophy" with sul-cal enlargement, or images of ventricular dilatation [Figure 3.30]. When no previous images are available for comparison with the ones obtained in the chronic stage, the correct interpretation and the es-tablishment of an adequate behavioral/anatomical correlation may not be possible.

Similar problems befall MR with images obtained with only one

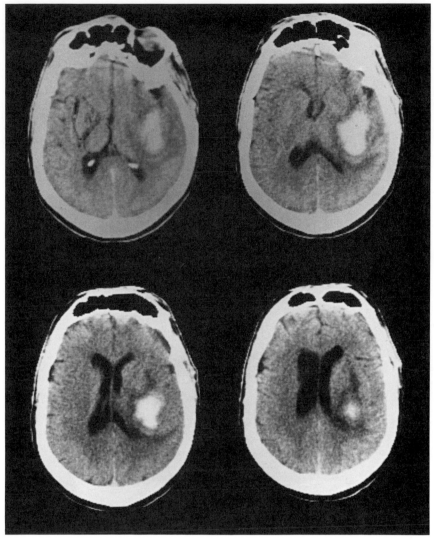

(B)

pulse sequence. For instance, it is known that T_1 weighted images
obtained with an Inversion Recovery pulse sequence (IR) provide
maximal anatomical detail. With this pulse sequence, however, infarctions appear as dark areas, in precisely the same range of grays
used to depict the ventricular system or any region filled with cerebrospinal fluid, such as the cerebral sulci and fissures. When infarcts
are small, and close to one of these structures, they may not be
readily distinguishable. T_2 weighted images obtained with Spin Echo

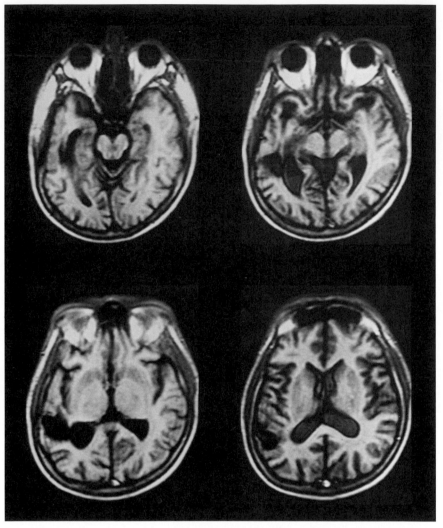

(A)

FIGURE 3.23. Chronic MRs of the two patients whose CTs are seen in Figure 3.22. The residual defect corresponding to the left hemisphere hematoma is rather large and occupies the posterior portion of the left-middle and superior temporal gyri (A). It involves both cortical and subcortical areas.

The defect resulting from the right hemisphere hematoma (B) involves the posterior insula, and resembles a knife-cut under the posterior portion of the temporal lobe. Otherwise, it leaves cortical structures intact. Thus, the lesion disconnects the posterior regions of the temporal lobe, as well as part of the inferior parietal lobule, but spares overlying cortices. Although in the acute and peri-acute stages there were striking similarities be-

pulse sequences (SE) show the damaged area as a region of intense bright signal, more easily distinguishable from the bright signals generated by white and even gray matter.

It should be emphasized that any meaningful relation between a given anatomical image and a particular neuropsychological pattern

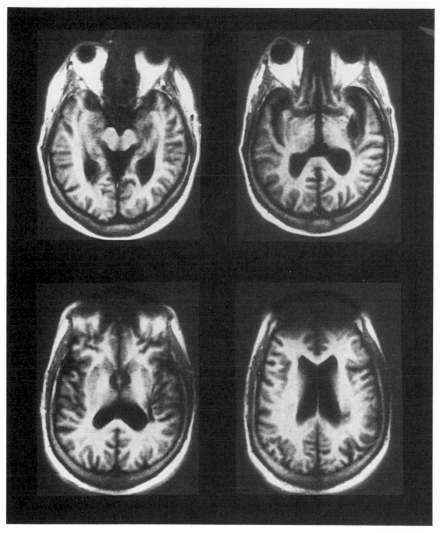

(B)

tween the lesions, the chronic images are entirely different from each other.

Patient A's residual defect was an aphasia, with fluent speech and frequent semantic paraphasias, which represents an improvement over his initial semantic jargon. At the time MR was obtained, formal language testing still revealed severely defective visual naming, impaired sentence and digit repetition, and abnormal comprehension of complex verbal material. This does represent an improvement over the acute clinical picture, that of a severe semantic jargon aphasia.

Patient B's residual deficit was impaired recognition of singing voices, impaired pitch recognition, and impaired pitch production in singing.

depends on a reasonable temporal closeness between the epoch at which the image and the neuropsychological data were obtained. As mentioned earlier, during the acute period, edema and distortion of brain structures often occur and it is not possible to define precisely the amount and location of destroyed tissue. When such im-

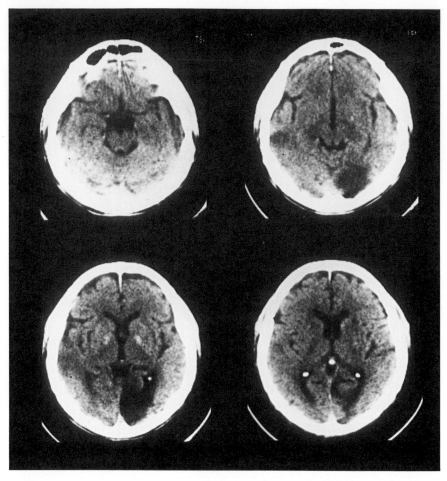

FIGURE 3.24. CT obtained less than 24 hours after a 75-year-old, right-handed man acutely developed a severe language impairment, characterized by perseverative paraphasic speech, a major deficit in aural comprehension, and a disturbance of visual naming and sentence repetition. The CT shows a well-defined area of decreased density in the right occipital lobe and an ill-defined lower-density area in the left temporal lobe.

The image in the right occipital region is that of an old infarct, which was not responsible for the new symptoms of the patient. These were due to a new cerebrovascular event, suggested radiologically by the faintly abnormal region in the left hemisphere.

The patient's past history did confirm the occurrence of a right occipital infarct several years before.

ages are related to observations made during the chronic state, the interpretation will be, of necessity, quite erroneous. Naturally, the same applies to the inverse situation, that is, relating the results of acute neuropsychological observation obtained in the acute state with anatomy derived from chronic images.

The most reliable anatomical and neuropsychological data are those obtained in the chronic stage. However, data obtained during the acute or periacute period are not necessarily useless. Provided early anatomical and neuropsychological observations coincide, their relations are still interpretable, and may be quite revealing. It is the cross-correlation of data from different epochs that is methodologically unacceptable.

Neuroanatomical Resolution

The limits of neuroanatomical resolution are set by the best of available technology. Current-generation CT scans define anatomical

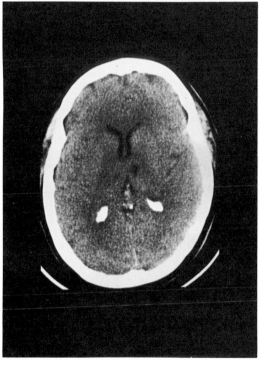

(A)

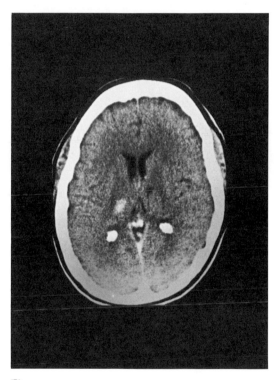

(B)

FIGURE 3.25. CT (A) of a 45-year-old, right-handed woman who acutely became confused and later developed somnolence, *right* hemiparesis, and hemisensory impairment. She was uncooperative for testing, but defects in naming and verbal comprehension were noted. Sentence repetition was normal. This CT, obtained in the first day of symptoms, shows a well-defined anterior thalamic infarct in the *right* hemisphere that could not account for the right-sided sensory-motor symptoms and was the unlikely cause of the language disturbance.

CT (B) of same patient obtained 12 days later. It reveals another and more recent infarct involving the left thalamus and part of the internal capsule. This infarct could certainly induce the sensory-motor defects mentioned above. The combination, in conjunction with the previous right thalamic infarction, may have contributed to the inaugural behavioral disturbance. This patient did *not* have a history of previous infarction.

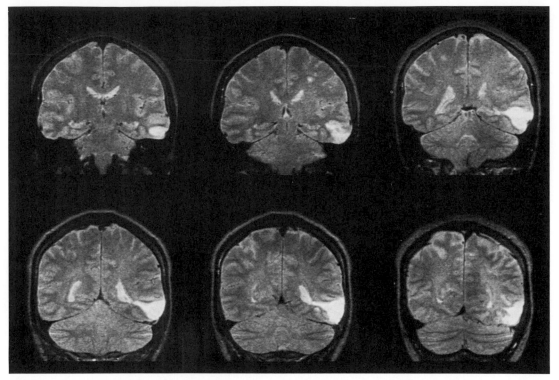

(A)

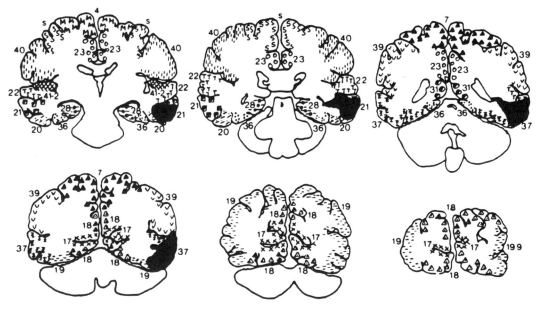

(B)

structures as small as 1 mm in the plane of section. For current-generation MR, structures as small as 1 mm on the plane of section can be well-visualized. From the point of view of microstructure, these by-now astounding *in vivo* resolutions are actually modest. After all, 1 mm of cortical surface subtends many cortical columns. However, from the perspective of cortical cytoarchitecture, or neurophysiologically defined cortical regions, a resolution of 1 mm to 2 mm is quite respectable. In relation to thalamic or basal ganglia nuclei, the resolution is equally impressive. The point is that current static imaging methodology visualizes neural structure at a level that permits the neuroanatomical definition of most nonmicroscopic lesions resulting from acquired neurological disease or neurosurgical ablations. It does not permit the direct visualization of cellular pathology. Naturally, it allows no visualization of dysfunctional states without structural pathology.

Neuroanatomical Description

We have already shown that CT and MR permit the study of the living brain's macrostructure with a degree of detail occasionally comparable to that obtained at post-mortem. On occasion, MR may actually provide more information than a post-mortem examination can, considering that it does permit multiple slicing of the same brain in varied incidences, something pathologists may dream of but cannot achieve. However, the analysis of CT and MR images poses special problems that go beyond the requisite knowledge of neuroanatomy. For a variety of technical reasons, the incidence of cuts varies from institution to institution, from patient to patient, and, often, in the same patient, from one scanning epoch to another. Whatever incidence is actually used, it poses special problems because the angle is likely to be remarkably different from that used in standard neuroanatomical sectioning at the anatomy table, thus yielding images that do not correspond directly to the depictions known from anatomical atlases. Such differences make it difficult to localize abnormal areas precisely. Frequently, they mislead the unalerted observer, who merely relies on a good eye for the anatomy. Although

FIGURE 3.26. Acute (four days after stroke) T_2 weighted MR images (A) and corresponding templates (B) of a 33-year-old, right-handed man who acutely developed a fluent aphasia, mildly paraphasic speech, and alexia. The patient was never agraphic, was always able to repeat, but had marked difficulties in specific name retrieval, which persisted even as other defects improved. The area of abnormally bright signal involves most of the middle and part of the inferior temporal gyri (all of lateral 37, as well as areas 21 and 20). It extends into the underlying white matter and reaches the ventricular wall at the level of the trigone.

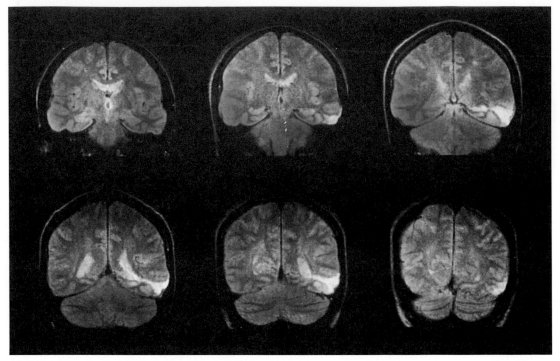

(A)

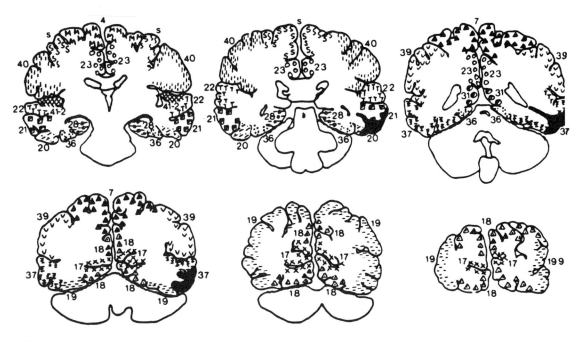

(B)

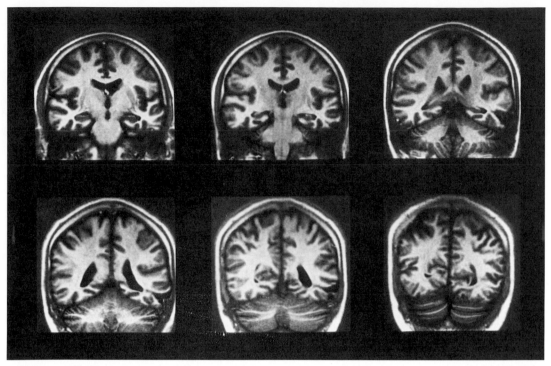

(C)

FIGURE 3.27. Chronic T_2 weighted MR images (A and B) of the patient in Figure 3.26. The area of abnormal bright signal is more restricted here, involving only a small portion of the middle and inferior temporal gyri (areas 21 and 20, and part of lateral 37). By the time this image was obtained, the patient had improved and had only a mild reading defect. His specific name retrieval difficulty persisted.

Chronic T_1 weighted MR images (C) of this patient obtained at the same time as the T_2 weighted image in (A). The low-signal area in these images delineates the actual region of destroyed brain substance. Note that the area is smaller than in the corresponding T_2 image.

this may not be critical for the clinician who simply wants to know about a lesion's nature and rough extent, the issue is vital for the scientist who wants to correlate lesion with dysfunction. Certainly, the comparison of successive scans in a given patient, or the comparison of images from several patients within a group, is not permissible under such circumstances. Even for the clinician, the rapid "eyeball" impressions can be misleading (see the example in Figure 4.13). In order to obviate these difficulties, we and others have developed systems of brain templates so as to constitute a virtual road map to localization of cortical lesions and help in the analyses of CT and MR images (Gado, Hanaway, & Frank, 1979; Kertesz, Harlock, & Coates, 1979; Luzzatti, Scotti, & Gattoni, 1979; Mazzocchi & Vig-

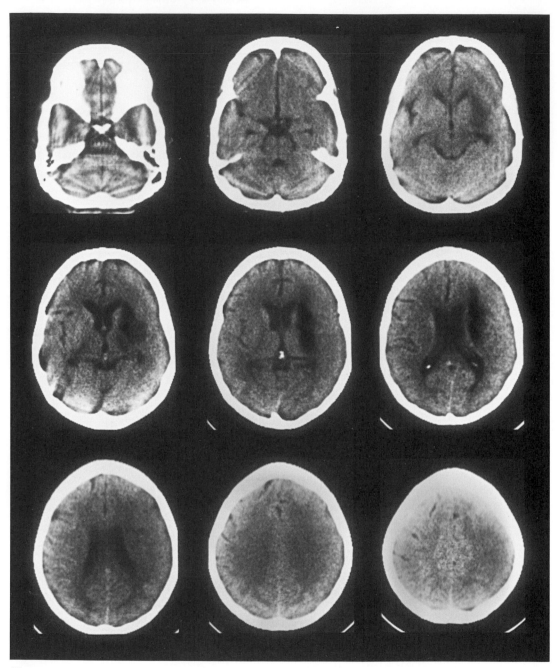

(A)

FIGURE 3.28. CT of the patient in Figure 2.12 obtained 11 days after the infarct occurred: (A) without contrast, (B) with contrast.

Note that in A, the only region of decreased density is in the basal ganglia. All the areas that previously showed decreased density are now isodense; that is, the damaged area has the same density as the surrounding normal tissue, absorbs radiation to the same degree, and is thus visually reconstructed with the same gray values. This effect might lead to the interpretation that the infarct was in the basal ganglia only and that the low density seen in the frontal, temporal, and parietal lobes in the first scan might have represented

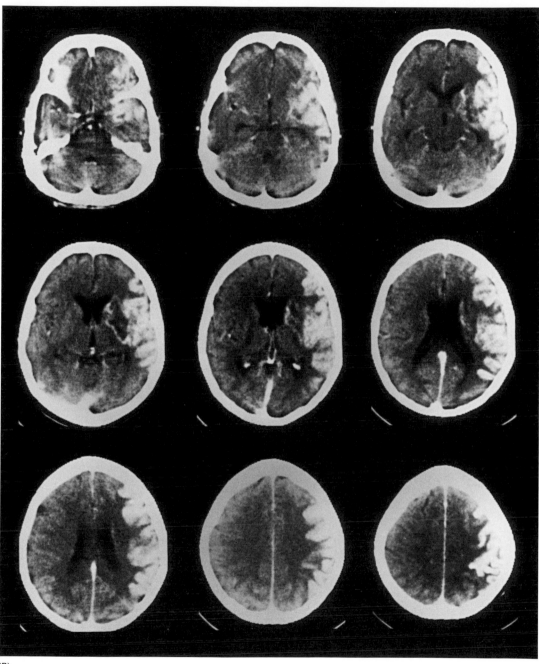

(B)

transient edema. Note, however, that in B, both the basal ganglia and the frontal, temporal, and parietal cortices reveal gray matter enhancement, a clear indication that the infarction involved not only the basal ganglia, but also those cortical regions.

Inspection of the unenhanced scan might easily have led to the erroneous conclusion that the symptoms (including the marked neglect and anosognosia, all of which still persisted at the time of this second scan), were due to a basal ganglia infarct alone.

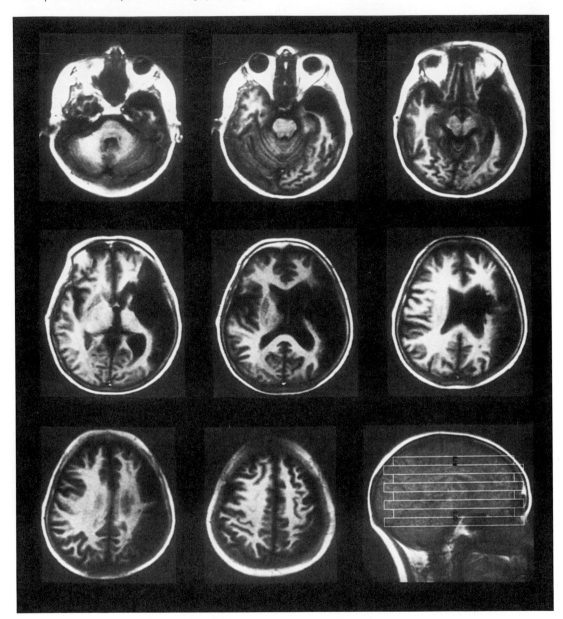

FIGURE 3.29. Chronic MR (T$_1$ weighted image) of the patient discussed in Figure 3.28. Note that the lesion involves not only the basal ganglia and internal capsule, but most of the territory of the right middle cerebral artery.

nolo, 1979; Naeser & Hayward, 1978; Poeck, de Blesser, & von Keyserlingk, 1984). In the following chapter we will describe our own method and discuss procedures for its use.

Neuroimaging of Cerebral Asymmetries and of the Ventricular System

Cerebral Asymmetries

The discovery of notable asymmetries in the region of the human auditory cortex (Geschwind & Levitsky, 1968) called attention to the possibility that an easily observable gross anatomical feature might provide an index of cerebral organization related to cognition. Geschwind noted that the planum temporale, the region of auditory association cortex (area 22) located immediately behind the primary auditory cortex (areas 41/42), is larger on the left than on the right in about 65% of human brains, by a factor as big as sevenfold. Because the region of the planum corresponds in great part to the so-called Wernicke's area, the possibility of a functional meaning to this asymmetry is quite compelling. Research over the past two decades has replicated Geschwind's findings and even demonstrated their early appearance during gestation (Chi, Dooling, & Gilles, 1977; Galaburda et al, 1978; Teszner et al, 1972; Wada, Clarkek, & Hamm, 1975; Witelson & Pallie, 1973). However, the hope that cerebral asymmetries would be unequivocal predicators of dominance for different psychological processes, or even a reliable correlate of handedness has not materialized yet (Chui & Damasio, 1980; Koff et al, 1986; LeMay, 1977). Nonetheless, the investigation of the meaning of cerebral asymmetries is far from over and it is important to note the presence or absence of asymmetries in the auditory system, especially when they are of large magnitude, and to search for the possibility of asymmetries of possible functional significance in other brain regions.

A standard method to study cerebral asymmetries in CT was described by Chui and Damasio (1980). In that study, neurologically normal subjects had their handedness assessed and received a CT without contrast. The scans were obtained at 15 degree angulation to the orbitomeatal line. The images were enlarged by approximately +80% of the original size, and asymmetry measurements were made at the lowest cut that showed both the frontal horns and the trigone region. The presence or absence of occipital and frontal petalias was also assessed. Petalias are virtually carvings of the inner surface of skull bones, visible in cross-section and traditionally studied in endocasts of skulls by anthropologists. Asymmetric petalias are direct indicators of asymmetric hemisphere sizes and shapes. In order to study petalias, to assess occipital and frontal width asym-

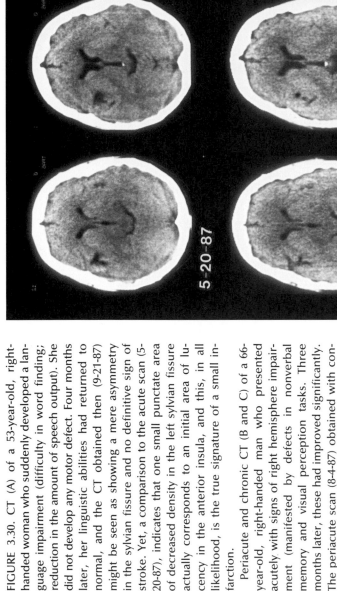

5-20-87

9-21-87

(A)

FIGURE 3.30. CT (A) of a 53-year-old, right-handed woman who suddenly developed a language impairment (difficulty in word finding; reduction in the amount of speech output). She did not develop any motor defect. Four months later, her linguistic abilities had returned to normal, and the CT obtained then (9-21-87) might be seen as showing a mere asymmetry in the sylvian fissure and no definitive sign of stroke. Yet, a comparison to the acute scan (5-20-87), indicates that one small punctate area of decreased density in the left sylvian fissure actually corresponds to an initial area of lucency in the anterior insula, and this, in all likelihood, is the true signature of a small infarction.

Periacute and chronic CT (B and C) of a 66-year-old, right-handed man who presented acutely with signs of right hemisphere impairment (manifested by defects in nonverbal memory and visual perception tasks. Three months later, these had improved significantly. The periacute scan (8-4-87) obtained with contrast enhancement shows areas of increased density in the right frontal lobe, clearly seen in cuts 2, 3, and 4. the chronic scan (11-19-87) does show an area of decreased density (cut 3), which corresponds to the old stroke. The interpretation of the abnormal image seen in the next cut cannot be that of a mere enlarged sulcus. However, in cuts 1 and 2, the images in the right frontal region might well be interpreted as only an enlarged sylvian fissure if it were not for the periacute evidence of cortical enhancement in the same region, which tells us that there was, in fact, an infarction at this level.

130

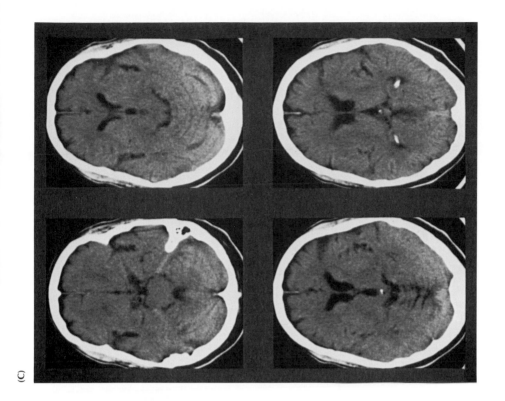

(C)

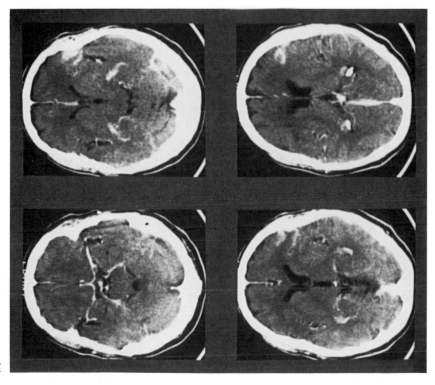

(B)

metry, and to determine the direction of the straight sinus, several steps were taken: (a) a line was drawn through the anterior sector of the falx, septum pellucidum, and pineal body; (b) perpendiculars to this sagittal line were drawn at the most anterior and posterior extents of the inner table, thus defining the antero-posterior (AP) diameter; (c) when these lines did not demarcate the points of maximum expansion of both hemispheres, parallel lines were traced, thus yielding the difference in length between the two hemispheres, both in the frontal and in the occipital region (the petalias); (d) additional parallel lines were drawn at two points on the AP line, at 16% and 90% of the entire AP diameter; and (e) the distance be-

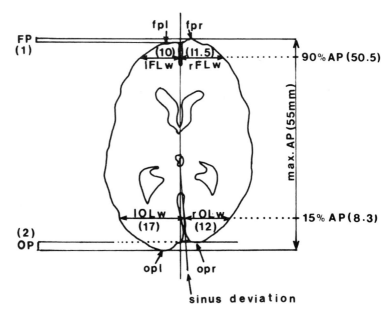

FIGURE 3.31. Line drawing of a CT cut used to measure occipital and frontal asymmetries. It exemplifies the procedure involved in the determination of occipital and frontal petalia, occipital and frontal width asymmetry, and deviation of the straight sinus.

Frontal Petalia:
$$FP = \frac{fpl - fpr}{fpl + fpr} \times 100 \quad \text{(in the example} = -1.8\%)$$

Occipital Petalia:
$$OP = \frac{opl - opr}{opl + opr} \times 100 \quad \text{(in the example} = +3.6\%)$$

Frontal Lobe Width:
$$FLW = \frac{lFLw - rFLw}{lFLw + rFLw} \times 100 \quad \text{(in the example} = -6.9\%)$$

Occipital Lobe Width:
$$OLw = \frac{lOLw - rOLw}{lOLw + rOLw} \times 100 \quad \text{(in the example} = +17.3\%)$$

tween the sagittal line and the inner table at these points was compared between the sides, thus giving the frontal and occipital symmetry.

Figure 3.31 depicts a slight modification of this method as currently used in our laboratory.

The overall CT asymmetry pattern seen in Chui and Damasio's subjects confirmed the previous findings (LeMay, 1976), that is, that the left occipital lobe was more often longer and wider than the right, and that the reverse was true for the frontal lobe. However, the trend for posterior regions to be larger in the left hemisphere than in the right was not correlated with hand preference.

The method just described aims at detecting indirect signs of the language cortex asymmetries noted by Geschwind. Although there is some evidence that a few of the imaging measures correlate with the auditory asymmetries as seen at autopsy (Pieniadz & Naeser, 1984), a direct analysis of the auditory region, especially of the critical planum temporale, must be the ideal approach to the issue. MR may provide the right venue, although a workable and reliable method has not been developed yet. For instance, it has not yet been determined if the CT technique just described to measure asymmetries in the length and width of the posterior regions is directly applicable to MR. MR cuts are usually obtained closer to the orbitomeatal line, and, on occasion, even with negative tilts. The cuts that show both the frontal horns and the trigone generally cut through a higher region of the occipital lobe. Even so, preliminary results seem to indicate that the direction of the asymmetry in both MR and CT is the same. However, the magnitude of the difference may vary considerably from case to case. Figure 3.32 shows a set of comparisons of results in the same patient based on CT and MR.

The use of parasagittal cuts permits the visualization of the sylvian fissure, and allows the confirmation of the observations of Rubens, Mahowald, and Hutton (1976) on its asymmetric course. [Figure 3.33]. Sequential coronal cuts show that the posterior end of the sylvian fissure is lower and extends more posteriorly in the left hemisphere, confirming the angiographic findings of LeMay and Culebras (1972) [see Figure 3.34].

Ventricular System

It is always important to analyze the state of the ventricular system in neuroimages because of these structures' landmark value. The shape and size of ventricular chambers are often modified by focal lesions, not only by those in the vicinity, but also by those in the cortex and white matter, which are often far removed. In general, this mechanical effect is due to (a) pushing on the ventricular walls by tumors or edema, (b) pulling and stretching of the ventricular

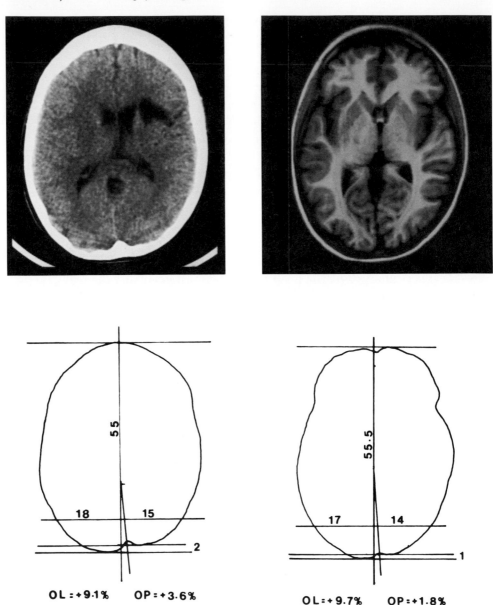

(Patient A)   OL : +9.1%   OP : +3.6%

OL: +9.7%   OP: +1.8%

FIGURE 3.32. Two examples of pairs of CT and MR cuts of the same patients with measurements of occipital asymmetries. The direction of the asymmetry is the same, but the magnitude of the difference is quite varied. This is most probably the result of the cuts' different angulation. In some MR scans, it is not possible to use this method because of the negative angulation of the cuts. In Patient (A) both the CT and MR show a left occipital petalia (OP) and a larger left occipital lobe (OL).

In Patient (B) both CT and MR show a reversal of the occipital asymmetry with a larger right occipital lobe (OL has negative value) and no petalia.

In CT, the tracing of the brain area is done at the inner table of the skull. Because MR does not visualize bone structures, the outer limit of the brain is used instead.

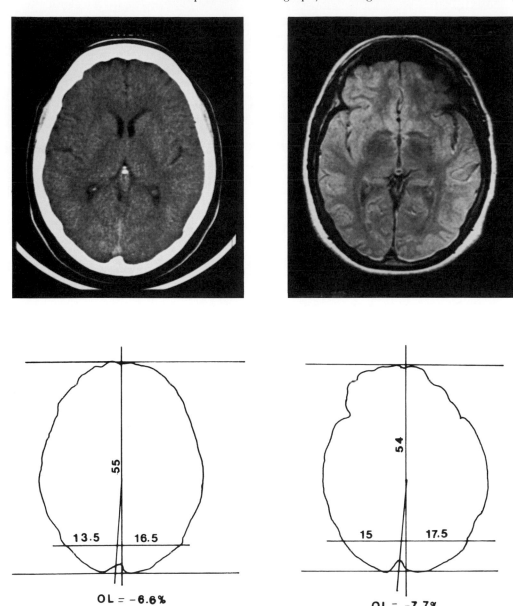

OL = -6.6%

OL = -7.7%

(Patient B)

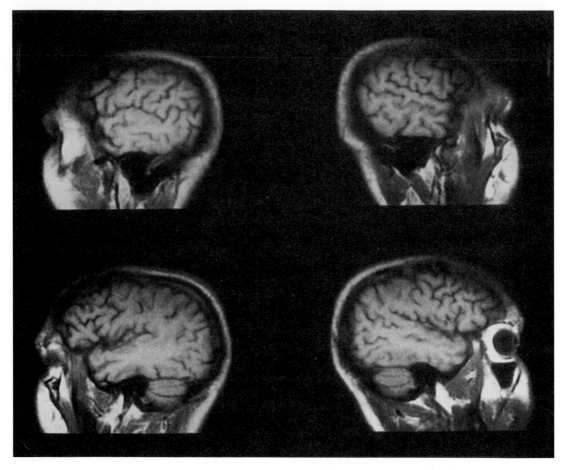

FIGURE 3.33. Parasagittal T₁ weighted MR images of both hemispheres of one patient, a right-handed subject. The left hemisphere is on the left-hand side, the right on the right. The upper two cuts represent the most tangential cuts showing the course of the sylvian fissure. Note that in the left hemisphere (left side of the figure) the sylvian fissure has a more horizontal and longer course than on the right.

walls during the repair phase of infarctions, or (c) increased intraventricular pressure, as in hydrocephalus. Ventricular size can also be reduced, as a result of increased pressure from the surrounding cerebral parenchyma, as is often found in head injury and pseudotumor cerebri. All of these modifications can be described qualitatively and charted accordingly.

In degenerative cerebral diseases, such as Alzheimer's disease or Huntington's disease, which may occur independently or in combination with a stroke or a tumor, the changes in ventricular shape and size are often subtle and the decision as to whether or not they are present may have to rely on a quantitative method. We have

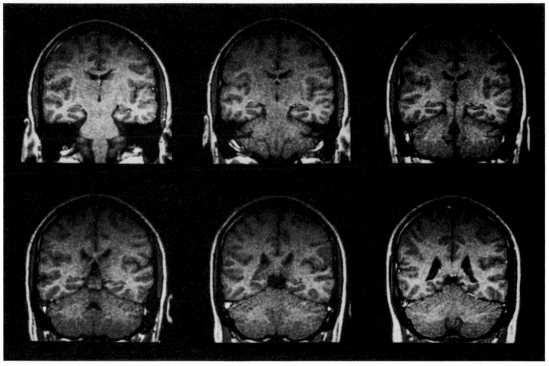

(A)

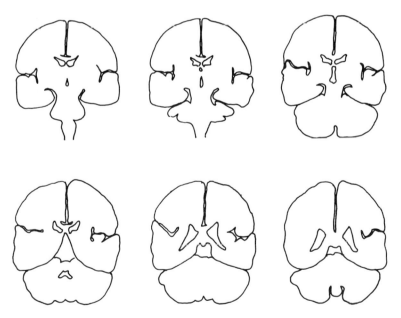

(B)

FIGURE 3.34. Coronal T_1 weighted MR images of a normal right-handed subject (A). Note that in the last cuts, the left sylvian fissure (seen on the right) is placed lower than the one on the right (left-hand side). And, it is still possible to see it clearly in the very last cut, while the right sylvian fissure is no longer present at that level. The line drawing of the MR cuts (B) highlights the sylvian fissure.

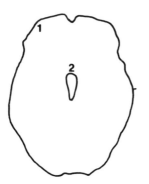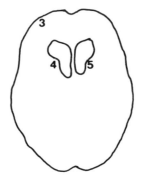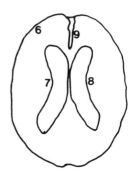

FIGURE 3.35. Illustration of the technique used for ventricular measurements as described by H. Damasio et al, 1983. Cuts 4, 5, and 7 of the CT of the patient in Figure 3.2 were used for the diagrams. The numbers refer to the curves delineating the surface subtended (a) by the brain, and (b) by the ventricular structures, at each level.

The measurement of the third ventrical is determined on cut 4, as a ratio between the area of 2 and 1; the measurement of the frontal horns is made on cut 5, as the ratio between the sum of areas 4 plus 5, and area 3; the body of ventricle, on cut 7, as the ratio between the sum of areas 7 plus 8, and 6; the measurement of the interhemispheric fissure is determined on the same cut as the body of the lateral ventrical, from the ratio between the areas of curves 9 and 6.

described one method to perform such a quantitative analysis (H. Damasio et al, 1983).

In that study we determined the area occupied by (a) the frontal horns, (b) the body of the lateral ventricles, (c) the third ventricle, and (d) the anterior interhemispheric fissure. We expressed it as a ratio to the area of the whole brain within the slice in which the structures were measured. Such measurements were carried out in an entirely normal elderly population. The subjects had been screened for neurological disorders and for neuropsychological deficits. Comparisons were made to groups of patients with varied types of dementia. We found that the ventricular/brain ratios and the interhemispheric tissue/brain ratios provided a powerful means to discriminate between normal and demented subjects at an overall level of accuracy of 77% [See Figure 3.35].

In conclusion, CT and MR are powerful technologies that permit the detection of neuropathological conditions and the comprehensive assessment of varied aspects of the injured brain's neuroanatomical status. There are limits, however, to anatomical resolution and pathological detection, and not all specimens or epochs postonset of brain damage lend themselves to optimal study of neuroanatomy.

References

Anderson SW, Damasio A, Damasio H: Troubled letters but *not* numbers: Domain-specific cognitive impairments following focal damage in frontal cortex, to be published.

Anderson SW, Damasio H, Tranel D: The use of tumor and stroke patients in neuropsychological research: A methodological critique. *Journal of Clinical and Experimental Neuropsychology* **10**:32, 1988.

Chase TN, Foster NL, Fedio P, Brooks R, Mansi L, DeChiro G: Regional cortical dysfunction in Alzheimer's disease as determined by positron emission tomography. *Annals of Neurology* **15**(suppl): S170–S174, 1984.

Chi JG, Dooling EC, Gilles FH: Left-right asymmetries of the temporal speech areas of the human fetus. *Archives of Neurology* **34**:346–348, 1977.

Chui H, Damasio A: Human cerebral asymmetries evaluated by computed tomography. *Journal of Neurology, Neurosurgery, and Psychiatry* **43**:873–878, 1980.

Damasio A: The brain binds entities and events by multiregional activation from convergence zones. *Neural Computation* **1**:123–132, 1989a.

Damasio A: Multiregional co-attended retroactivation: A new model of the neural substrates of cognition, *Cognition* 1989b.

Damasio A, Damasio H: The anatomical basis of pure alexia. *Neurology* **33**:1573–1583, 1983.

Damasio H, Eslinger P, Damasio A, Rizzo M, Huang H, Demeter S: Quantitative computed tomographic analysis in the diagnosis of dementia. *Archives of Neurology* **40**:715–719, 1983.

Escourolle R, Poirier J: *Manual of Basic Neuropathology*. Philadelphia, W. B. Saunders, 1978.

Eslinger P, Damasio AR: Severe cognitive disturbance of higher cognition after bilateral frontal lobe ablation. *Neurology* **35**:1731–1741, 1985.

Foster NL, Chase TN, Mansi L, Brooks R, Fedio P, Patronas NJ, DiChiro G: Cortical abnormalities in Alzheimer's disease. *Annals of Neurology* **16**:649–654, 1984.

Fox P, Perlmutter J, Raichle M: A stereotactic method of anatomical localization for positron emission tomography. *Journal of Computer Assisted Tomography* **9**(1):141–153, 1985.

Friedland RP, Budinger TF, Ganz E, Yano Y, Mathis CA, Koss B, Ober BA, Heusman RH, Derenzo SE: Regional cerebral metabolic alterations in dementia of the Alzheimer type: Positron emission tomography with 18-F fluorodeoxyglucose. *Journal of Computer Assisted Tomography* **7**(4):590–598, 1983.

Gado M, Hanaway J, Frank R: Functional anatomy of the cerebral cortex by computed tomography. *Journal of Computerized Axial Tomography* **3**:1–19, 1979.

Galaburda AM, LeMay M, Kemper TL, Geschwind N: Right-left asymmetries in the brain. *Science* **199**:852–856, 1978.

Geschwind N, Levitsky W: Human brain: Left-right asymmetries in temporal speech region. *Science* **161**:186–187, 1968.

Graff-Radford N, Hyman B, Hart M, Damasio H, Tranel D, Rezai K, Van Hoesen GW, Damasio, A: Progressive anomia caused by Pick's disease: Involvement of left anterior temporal lobe, to be published.

Hyman BT, Damasio AR, Van Hoesen GW, Barnes CL: Alzheimer's disease: Cell specific pathology isolates the hippocampal formation. *Science* **225**:1168–1170, 1984.

Hyman BT, Van Hoesen GW, Kromer LJ, Damasio AR: Perforant pathway changes and the memory impairment of Alzheimer's disease. *Annals of Neurology* **20:**473–482, 1986.

Kertesz A, Harlock W, Coates R: Computer tomographic localization, lesion size, and prognosis in aphasia and nonverbal impairment. *Brain and Language* **8:**34–50, 1979.

Koff E, Naeser M, Pieniadz J, Foundas A, Levine H: Computer tomographic scan hemispheric asymmetries in right- and left-handed male and female subjects. *Archives of Neurology* **43:**487–491, 1986.

LeMay M: Morphological cerebral asymmetries of modern man, fossil man, and non-human primates. *Annals of the New York Academy of Science* **280:**349–366, 1976.

LeMay M: Asymmetries of the skull and handedness. *Journal of Neurological Sciences* **32:**243–253, 1977.

LeMay M, Culebras A: Human brain—Morphological differences in the hemispheres demonstrable by carotid arteriography. *New England Journal of Medicine* **287:**168–170, 1972.

Luzzatti C, Scotti G, Gattoni A: Further suggestions for cerebral CT localization. *Cortex* **15:**483–490, 1979.

Mazzocchi F, Vignolo LA: Localization of lesions of aphasia: Clinical CT scan correlations in stroke patients. *Cortex* **15:**627–654, 1979.

Naeser MA, Hayward RW: Lesion localization in aphasia with cranial computed tomography and the Boston Diagnostic Aphasia Exam. *Neurology* **28:**545–551, 1978.

Pieniadz J, Naeser M: Computed tomographic scan cerebral asymmetries and morphologic brain asymmetries—Correlation in the same cases postmortem. *Archives of Neurology* **41:**403–409, 1984.

Poeck K, de Bleser R, von Keyserlingk DG: Computed tomography localization of standard aphasic syndromes. *Advances in Neurology* **42:**71–89, 1984.

Rezai K, Damasio H, Graff-Radford N, Eslinger P, Kirchner P: Regional cerebral blood flow abnormalities in Alzheimer's disease. *Journal of Nuclear Medicine* **26**(5):105, 1985.

Rubens AB, Mahowald MW, Hutton JT: Asymmetry of the lateral (sylvian) fissures in man. *Neurology* **26:**620–624, 1976.

Talairach J, Szikla G: *Atlas d'anatomie stéréotaxique du télencéphale.* Paris, Masson et Cie, 1967.

Teszner D, Tzavaras A, Gruner J, Hécaen H.: L'asymetrie droite-gauche du planum temporale; A propos de l'étude anatomique de 100 cerveaux. *Revue Neurologique* **126:**444–449, 1972.

Wada JA, Clarkek R, Hamm A: Cerebral hemispheric asymmetry in humans: Cortical speech zones in 100 adult and 100 infant brains. *Archives of Neurology* **32:**239–246, 1975.

Witelson S, Pallie W: Left hemisphere specialisation for language in the newborn: Neuroanatomical evidence of asymmetry. *Brain:* **96:**641–646, 1973.

4

ROAD MAPS
TO NEUROANATOMY

The Development of Standard Templates

Because of the variability of angles of incidence in CT and MR, it became necessary to develop a system of brain templates that might serve as a virtual road map to localization of cortical lesions as they are seen in these scans. Most often, CT is obtained in relation to the inferior orbitomeatal line, with angulations varying between 10 degrees and 30 degrees. MR is generally obtained parallel to the orbitomeatal line and at a 90 degree angle (the coronal cuts). Thus, the first step in development of this method was to prepare different sets of templates, each with a different angulation in relation to the inferior orbitomeatal line. The chosen angles correspond to those most frequently used, ranging from 0 degrees to 90 degrees. The following procedure was used.

1. We obtained photographs of the lateral and mesial views of normal human brains.
2. On those photographs we marked the major cytoarchitectonic areas according to the classic cytoarchitectonic maps of Brodmann (1909), as well as to more recent maps of Sarkissow et al (1955) and Braak (1978).
3. The incidence and level of the CT cuts were also marked on the lateral and mesial surfaces of the brain, using the method described by Matsui and Hirano (1978) [Figures 4.1A & 4.1B].
4. The brain was then cut at the levels drawn in the photograph,

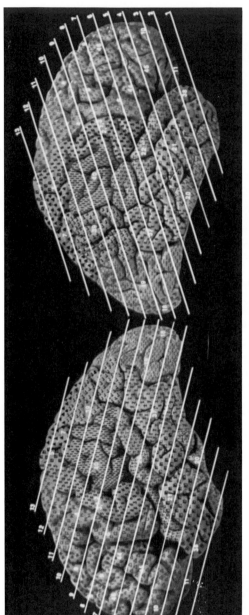

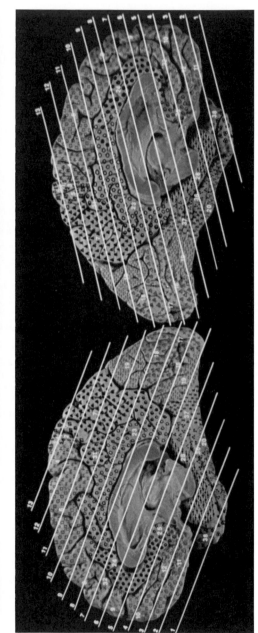

(A)

(B)

FIGURE 4.1. Lateral (A) and mesial (B) views of a brain, with markings corresponding to Brodmann's cytoarchitectonic areas. Lines 1 through 13 correspond to the level and incidence in which this particular brain was sectioned. The lines were marked according to the method described by Matsui and Hirano, with a 15 degree caudal angulation in relation to the inferior orbitomeatal line.

and the upper surface of the sections so obtained [Figure 4.2A] was used to chart a series of templates.

5. The cytoarchitectonic areas were marked in those templates, using as guidelines the previously obtained picture of the brain's lateral and mesial surface [Figure 4.2B].

Using this procedure, along with anatomical information available in standard atlases (DeArmond, Fusco, & Dewey, 1976; Hanaway, Scott, & Strother, 1977; Matsui & Hirano, 1978; Palacios, Fine, & Henghton, 1980; Schnitzlein & Murtagh, 1985), we prepared a total of six sets of templates covering incidence ranges of 0 degrees to 90 degrees (see Appendix).

To develop templates for the analysis of vascular territories, we plotted the boundaries of those territories, based on current knowledge of vascular anatomy (Lazorthes, Gouaze & Salamon, 1976; Salamon & Huang, 1976; Waddington, 1974), on the pre-existing template (Damasio, 1983, 1987) (see Appendix). Figure 4.3 represents an axial view of the thalamus with a more detailed subdivision of its perforating vessels.

Standard Procedure for the Analysis of CT and MR Images

A technician collects all the film transparencies obtained in a given case and masks the subject identification in all of them, substituting a numerical entry code on the basis of which imaging data are stored in both computer and hard-copy files. These steps ensure that the anatomical investigators are blind to the neurological and behavioral data collected in the same subject.

Working at a light table dedicated to charting, the investigators then proceed to:

1. In the case of CT, determine the angle of incidence in which tomographic cuts were obtained on the basis of a pilot scan and of the relative position of anatomical, cerebral, and bone landmarks.
2. In the case of MR, make the same determination on the basis of a midsagittal pilot cut. MR images do not show bone landmarks but their resolution is such that actual anatomical structures, for example, sulci, gyri, and visually recognizable gray matter structures, can be clearly identified.
3. Choose the set of best-fitting templates on the basis of the above determination.
4. Chart the lesion on the templates, at every level at which it occurs, using an X/Y plotting approach [Figures 4.4A, 4.4B, 4.5].
5. Superimpose over the template an appropriate "in-register"

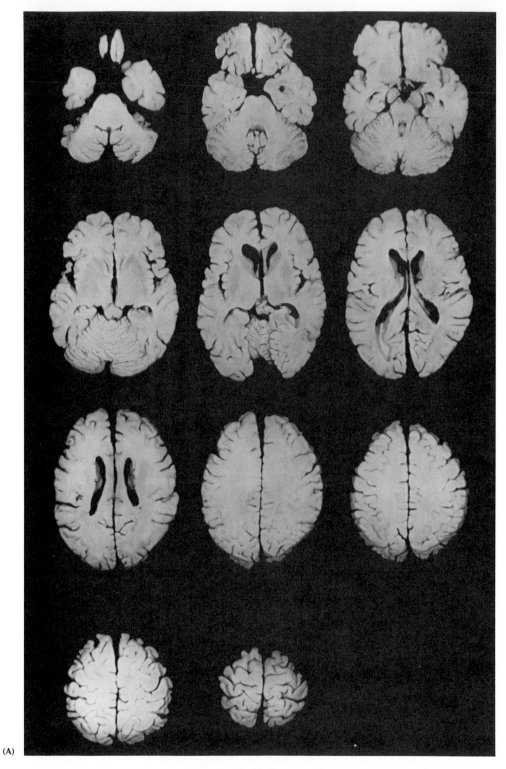

FIGURE 4.2. (A) Upper surface photographs of 11 of the sections obtained from the cutting of the brain seen in Figure 4.1. (B) Line drawings of those same sections. The numbers indicate the Brodmann's cytoarchitectonic areas that occur at each section.

144

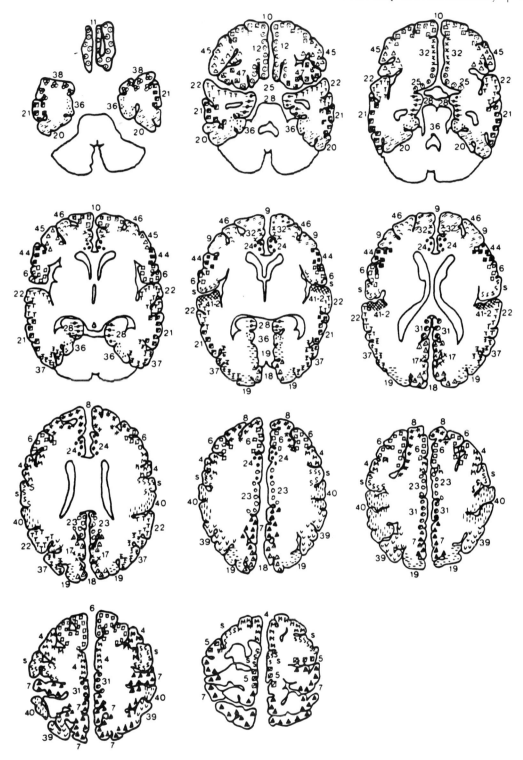

(B)

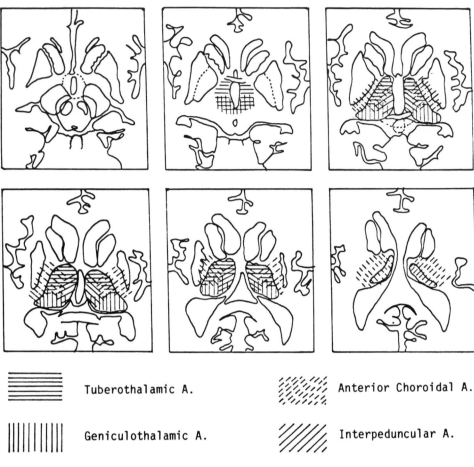

▤	Tuberothalamic A.	◨	Anterior Choroidal A.
▥	Geniculothalamic A.	◩	Interpeduncular A.

FIGURE 4.3. Thin-cut templates through the thalamus, in transverse view, with markings corresponding to the territories supplied by the different perforating thalamic vessels. (Reproduced with permission from Graff-Radford et al, *Brain* 108:485–516, 1985.)

transparency that contains anatomical cells representing neural "areas of interest" in both gray and white matter structures. (Each of those cells is limited by a linear boundary and has a letter and number code on the basis of which it can be anatomically identified [Figure 4.6A]).

6. Assign the area of damage charted in the template to the cells that encompass the abnormal images.

7. Estimate the amount of involvement within target cells. (Coded as 0 when less than 25% involvement of the total area is noted, 1 if the involvement is between 25% and 75%, and 2 if more than 75% of the total area is damaged.) This step can be

achieved in two ways: either use (a) a transparent square grid, count the number of units involved by the lesion at each level, and calculate the percentage in relation to the total number of units encompassed by each area of interest (which is the sum of units occupied by the region at each template level); or (b) transfer the template system into computer software, tracing the lesion's limits as marked on the template with a digitizer, followed by automated determination of the percentage of area involved.

8. Determine the vascular territory in which the lesion occurred, using the appropriate vascular transparency [Figure 4.6B].

9. Fill in the results of the previous analysis as a hard-copy visual record and a computerized record, keyed to the codes mentioned (see Appendix).

Some cerebral areas, for instance the occipital cortices, pose special localization problems and require the use of additional sets of cuts, generally coronal, and the appropriate charting of the cuts.

It should be noted that the number of cuts in the scan and in the correctly chosen set of templates may not coincide, for two reasons: varied thickness of cuts and individual brain size variations. The investigator, therefore, must search for the most appropriate scan/template matches, on a cut-by-cut basis, using all available anatomical constants, for example, ventricular system and prominent sulci [Figure 4.7]. Fortunately, current MR resolution provides such a wealth of landmarks that finding appropriate correspondences is no longer a daunting task.

The correspondences previously indicated are also a necessary complement to the X/Y plotting approach. In other words, X/Y plotting should be accompanied always by a counterchecking of the lesion plot in relation to identifiable landmarks. Although in most instances mere plotting will place the lesion accurately (the procedure and an instance of accurate plotting are given in Figure 4.5), in some instances, "blind" plotting may produce an inaccurate chart [see Figure 4.8]. This is why we do not advocate the use of fully automated analysis of lesions, although automation is theoretically possible with current computer technology. To make the contour of a CT or MR brain cut fit the contour of an idealized brain section is to court error.

Analysis of dynamic scans, PET, or SPET is a far more difficult task. The main reason for the added difficulty is that neither method provides sufficient anatomical detail.

Some automated PET analysis methods have been developed based on procedures for stereotactic localization of brain structures. However, stereotactic techniques have been largely established for the

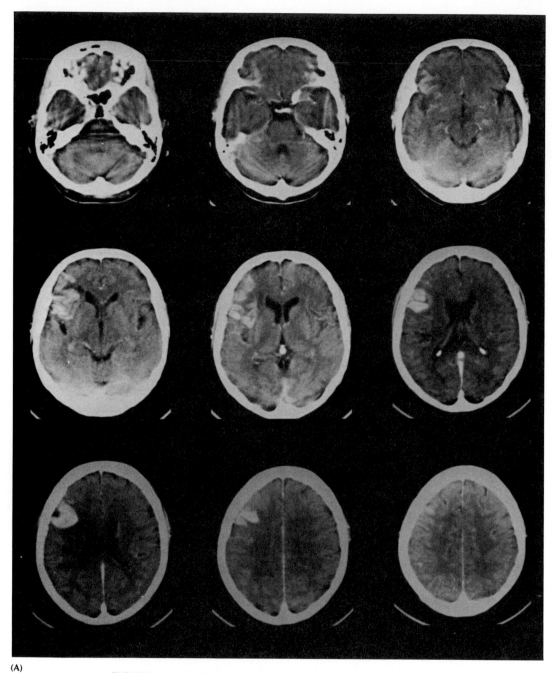

(A)

FIGURE 4.4. (A) Contrast-enhanced CT obtained in the second week post-stroke in a patient with aphasia of the Broca type.

  (B) Lesion seen in (A), in the left frontal lobe, transposed to the best-fitting template, using an X/Y proportional plotting approach.

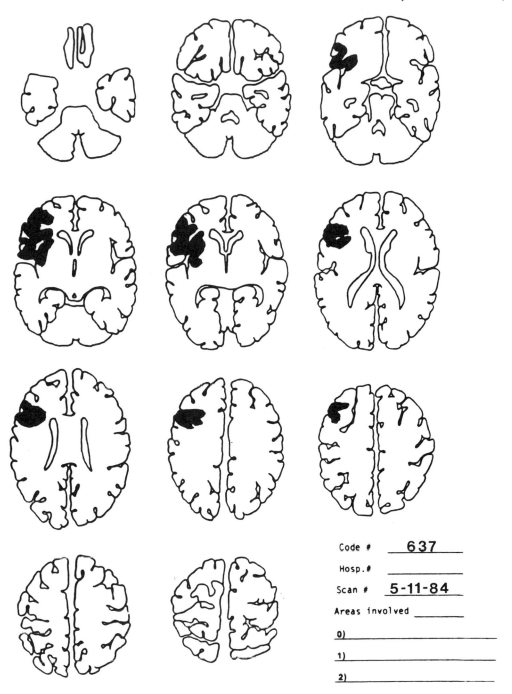

Code #   637

Hosp.#

Scan #   5-11-84

Areas involved

0)

1)

2)

(B)

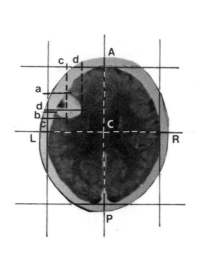

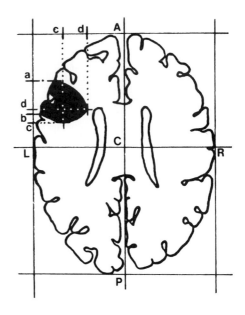

AP: 36 mm
C: 18 mm
LR: 30 mm

a: 7 mm / AP
b: 12 mm / AP
c: 13.5 mm / AP ; 5 mm / LR
d: 11.5 mm / AP ; 9 mm / LR

(A)

AP: 63 mm
C: 31.5 mm
LR: 48 mm

a: 12.3 mm
b. 21 mm
c: 23.6 mm ; 8 mm
d: 20.1 mm ; 14.4 mm

(B)

FIGURE 4.5. Demonstration of the X/Y proportional plotting approach.

(A)The CT cut is the actual size of the cut as seen on the CT film. There is an enhanced lesion in the left frontal lobe.

(B)Appropriate template cut, also in real size. By marking length (AP diameter) and width (LR diameter at the midpoint of the AP diameter) on both CT and template, the four points subtending the lesion in the CT (a, b, c, and d) can be transferred to the template.

deep gray structures of the basal ganglia and thalamus. There is some risk in applying to the cerebral cortex techniques developed for the deep gray areas, because cortical areas appear to be more affected by cerebral asymmetry and are perhaps more prone to individual variation. Be that as it may, a localization procedure based on stereotaxic references is shown in Figure 3.4 with a SPET study in a patient with Alzheimer's dementia. At the time SPET images were obtained, a lateral skull X-ray with radio-opaque markers was also obtained. The markers provide a reference for the patient's alignment in the scanner, and allowed us to mark in the skull X-ray both the incidence of cuts and the level at which each SPET cut was obtained. Talairach's quadrilatere (Talairach & Szikla, 1967) can then be superimposed on the skull X-ray, which will then permit the anatomical derivation of major cortical regions [Figure 3.4].

Another way to identify the anatomical location of areas of altered radiosignal is the integration of structural static information from CT or MR with the dynamic maps of SPET. The procedure is more cumbersome but also more accurate [Figure 3.5].

Sources of Error

The choice of a wrong template system is a major source of technical error that leads to incorrect anatomical placement of brain lesions. The first step towards a correct device of templates calls for the inspection of *all* cuts available, especially the lower cuts, which contain crucial landmarks for the determination of the incidence of a particular scan. In practical terms, it is necessary to compare the proportion of frontal lobe, temporal lobe, and posterior fossa structures as seen in the scan with those seen in the various template systems, and select the best match. It is not possible to choose the correct match based on the inspection of high cuts alone. In highlying cuts, the relation to anatomical constraints such as the ventricular system or bony landmarks is lost. Based on those few cuts, several template systems may appear appropriate, when, in fact, only one does fit. The following example illustrates the importance of this point.

A patient who suddenly developed a profound weakness of the left arm and whose reflexes in that extremity were slightly more active than in the normal limb had a CT that showed a right hemisphere lesion, predominantly supraventricular. Figure 4.9 shows the CT cuts in which the lesion can be seen. Based on those cuts alone, several template systems might be chosen, and, in fact, both a posterior fossa incidence as well as a near horizontal incidence seem equally appropriate. Yet the result of these two plottings yields completely different readings. Using the templates appropriate for a posterior fossa incidence, the lesion turns up in the parietal lobe and involves mainly the postrolandic gyrus and the anterior supramarginal gyrus. By contrast, with the other incidence, the lesion lands in the posterior frontal region, involving the precentral gyrus, a location that actually accords with the clinical picture. If attention would have been paid to the lower CT cuts [Figure 4.10], in which bony landmarks can be found demarcating the anterior, middle, and pos-

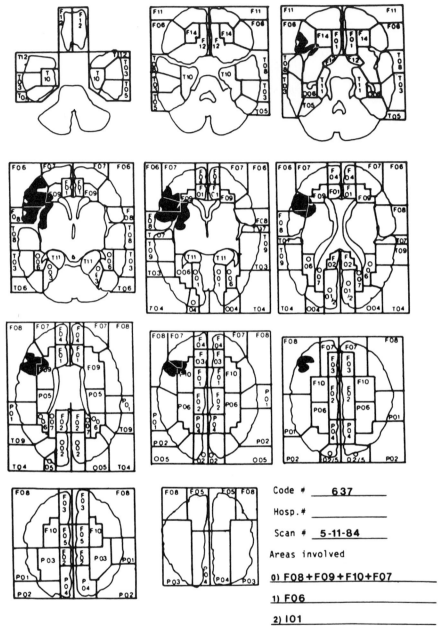

(A)

FIGURE 4.6. Same template as in Figure 4.4B with superimposed transparencies. (A) shows cell boundaries for the anatomical areas of interest, and (B) shows cell boundaries corresponding to vascular territories.

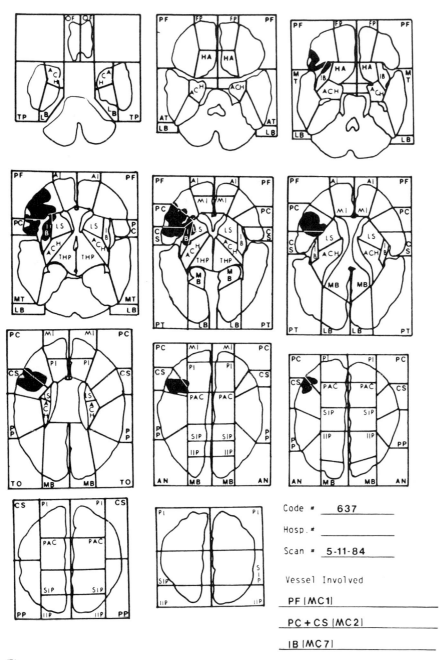

Code # _637_

Hosp. # _____

Scan # _5-11-84_

Vessel Involved

_PF (MC1)_

_PC + CS (MC2)_

_IB (MC7)_

(B)

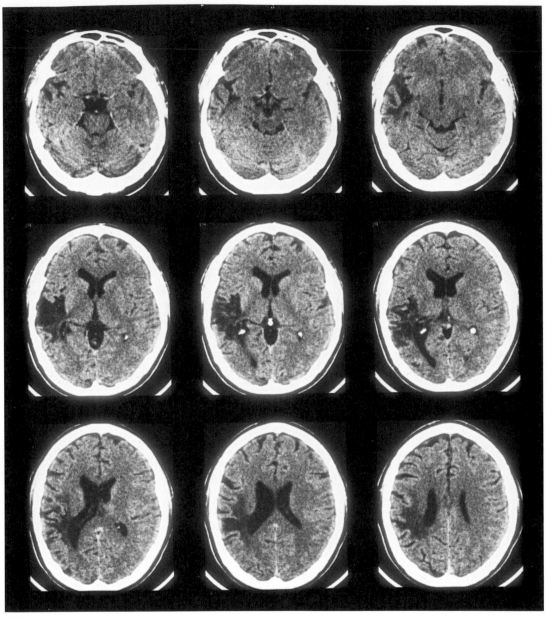

(A)

FIGURE 4.7. Chronic CT of a 49-year-old, right-handed man who five and one-half years earlier had become aphasic after a left hemispheric stroke. The aphasia was of the fluent type, with numerous phonemic paraphasic errors that the patient was aware of and tried to correct. Auditory comprehension was minimally impaired, but sentence repetition was quite defective. At the time of this CT, in spite of continued improvement, the patient was still unable to repeat sentences and still made frequent phonemic paraphasias.

This clinical profile conforms to the category of conduction aphasia and the lesion described below is one of two major types associated with this

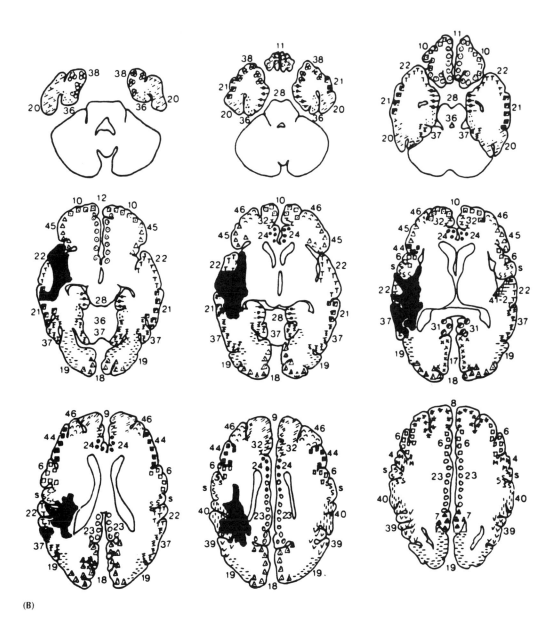

(B)

interesting aphasia type. Figure 2.16 shows the other major anatomical pattern seen in conduction aphasia.

The lesion involves the insula and superior temporal gyrus (auditory cortices and part of the surrounding area 22). It extends into the white matter underlying the inferior portion of the supramar-

ginal gyrus. It does not involve cortex of the inferior parietal lobule.

This CT (A) was obtained with thin (2-mm) cuts. The illustration shows only every third image of the full scan, but even so, the number of cuts on the appropriate template (B) set is far smaller. The plotting had to take this reduction into account. The CT in Figure 2.16 posed the same problem.

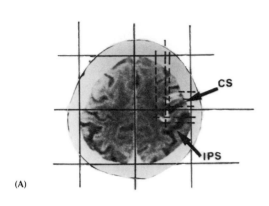

(A)

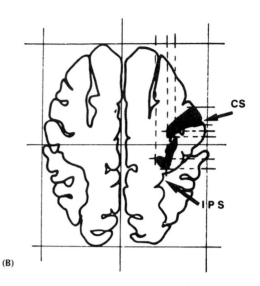

(B)

FIGURE 4.8. "Blind" X/Y plotting can be the source of errors. This figure illustrates the advantage of combining it with concurrent selection of the best-fitting template, making use of identifiable anatomical landmarks.

(A) CT cut showing the intraparietal sulcus (IPS) and the higher portion of the central sulcus (CS), immediately anterior to it. The same anatomical landmarks can be identified on the template (B).

(B) Using a "blind" X/Y plotting, the lesion would be plotted as involving most of the post-central gyrus, reaching all the way to the intraparietal sulcus.

(C)When the anatomical landmarks are taken into account, a more accurate plotting can be generated, showing the lesion to be in the prerolandic cortices (see Figure 4.9C).

terior fossae structures, instead of using only the upper half of the scan, *only* the more horizontal template system [Figure 4.9C] would have been chosen, and the proper localization would be immediately available. This is the only template system that shows the right proportion of frontal, temporal, and cerebellar structures.

Another example shows how two consecutive scans, a CT and an MR obtained in the same patient, may seem to depict lesions in different locations, again because attention was paid only to the cuts containing the lesion and not to the angle of scan. The CT was obtained in the first few days after the stroke and the lesion [Figure 4.11] was read, from correctly chosen templates, as being in the left frontal lobe just above Broca's area, mainly in the pre-motor region. However, superficial inspection of the MR obtained only a few days later [Figure 4.12], because of its entirely different incidence, suggested that the lesion was now in the parietal lobe. In fact, a plotting based only on the cuts in which the lesion is visualized would dislocate the lesion to the parietal cortices [Figure 4.12B]. When the appropriate steps are taken, the lesion is clearly in the same spot in both scans [see Figure 4.13 for the detailed description of the appropriate steps].

The proper analysis of this case was especially cumbersome because of the marked anterior tilt with which these MR images were obtained. Such a negative incidence is fortunately uncommon, but the steps necessary to deal with it, are presented in Figure 4.13. It is clear from this example that comparisons of studies obtained in the same patient, or in different patients in a group, must rely on appropriate template plottings if errors in anatomical interpretation are to be avoided.

Another example illustrates how, even for clinical understanding

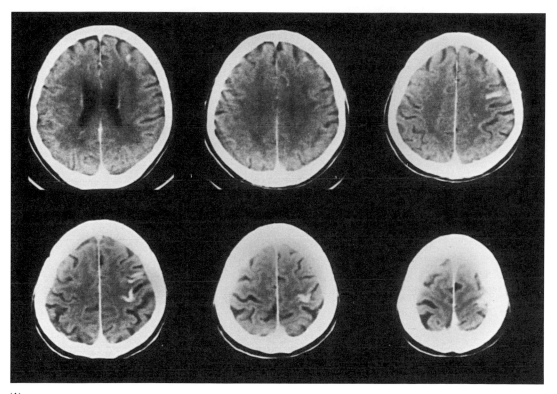

(A)

FIGURE 4.9. CT (A) of a patient with sudden monoparesis involving the left arm. Only the higher cuts, which show the are of damage, are represented. Given only these cuts, it would appear that *both* template systems shown here might be appropriate to chart the lesion. However, each of these template systems leads to an entirely different reading of the lesion's location. Using template (B), the lesion falls into the supramarginal gyrus and extends forward into part of the postrolandic gyrus. Using template (C), the lesion falls in the prerolandic gyrus. See Figure 4.10 for a means to resolve the problem.

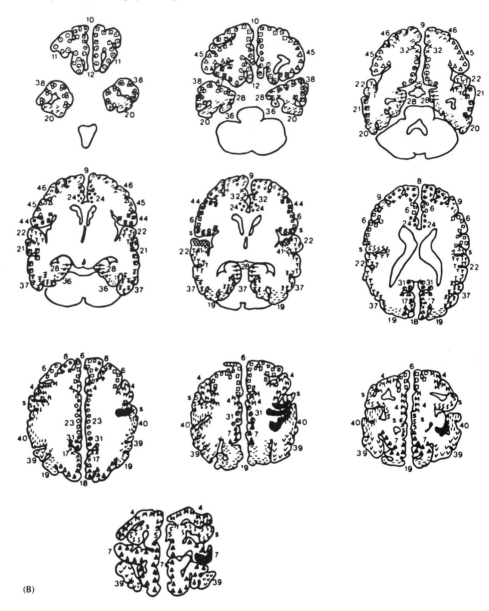

(B)

FIGURE 4.9. *continued.*

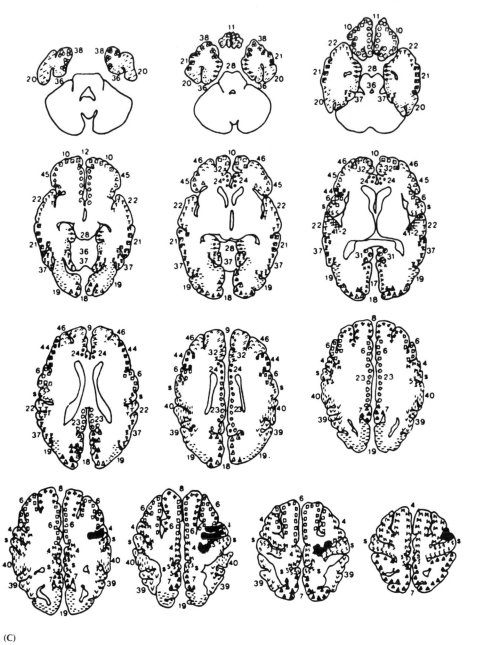

(C)

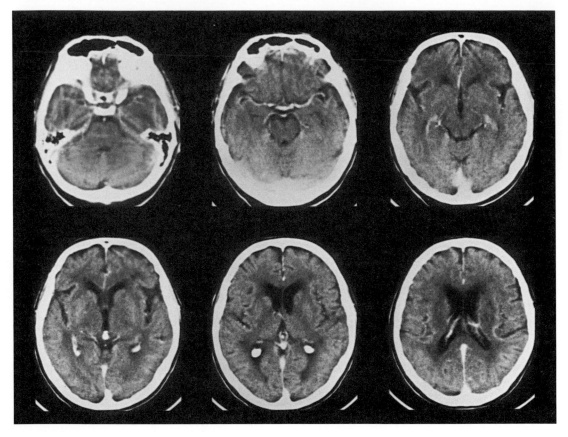

FIGURE 4.10. Lower cuts of the CT shown in Figure 4.9A. The proper inspection of *all* cuts, especially the lower ones, in which no abnormality is shown, makes it evident that only the template in Figure 4.9C fits the angulation of the CT, and is the only correct choice.

The steps critical to reach this decision are: (a) the careful inspection of the first two cuts, in which the relation between the amount of visible frontal and temporal lobe can be appreciated, and (b) the detection of the emergence of the occipital regions, which allows the choice of the correct template system by matching the lower cuts.

of neurological patients, a quick visual reading of a stroke image may lead to entirely wrong conclusions. Figure 4.14 shows a T_2 weighted MR of a patient who suddenly developed a right hemiparesis, more pronounced in the lower extremity than in the upper limb, and sparing both the hand and the face. The MR reading revealed an alleged occipital lobe infarct, a finding deemed unrelated to the hemiparesis. Unfortunately, it also revealed a small left basal ganglia lesion that was then thought to cause the motor defect. The proper reading of the MR, however, would have shown that the apparently posterior infarct was not in the occipital lobe, but, rather, in the mesial motor region, with an extension into the cingulate gyrus and into the deep white matter of the centrum semiovale. A lesion in this location should certainly cause a marked hemiparesis in the lower right limb, and its extension into the white matter might well undercut some descending fibers from the motor region of the upper limb and probably spare those from the hand and face region. On the other hand, the left basal ganglia lesion appears to be an old lacune in the mesial portion of the head of the caudate, a typical location for a "silent" lacune, and a lesion unlikely to cause the motor deficits described in this patient. Figure 4.15 shows a CT obtained a few days later in which, because of a different incidence, the localization was more straightforward.

Problem Areas for Charting

Because of anatomical configuration, some cerebral areas pose special charting problems. The occipital areas are a case in point. It is always important to decide if a lesion is above or below the calcarine fissure. However, the position of the calcarine fissure is not only variable from person to person but, in the same subject, it may be different in each hemisphere [Figure 4.16]. Furthermore, in transverse CT cuts, or even MR cuts, it is not possible to recognize the calcarine fissure. With MR, however, this problem can be solved by studying coronal cuts through the occipital lobe. As can be seen in Figure 4.17, the calcarine fissure is easily identified and permits the correct localization of lesions in relation to this anatomical structure.

When coronal cuts are read in an anteroposterior sequence, the first anatomical structure to be noted is the most anterior and inferior portion of the parieto-occipital sulcus as it is joined by the calcarine fissure. This provides a very typical image of a V placed sideways (<) with its vertex pointing towards the mesial surface of the hemisphere. In subsequent cuts, the two arms of the V get further and further apart. The superior arm, which corresponds to the parieto-occipital sulcus, "moves" superiorly; the inferior arm, the calcarine fissure, "moves" downward. Additional help in interpreting the coronal images can be afforded by a midsagittal cut showing the mesial view of hemisphere and revealing a direct image of these two sulci.

As can be seen by comparing transverse and coronal images in a case of infracalcarine infarct, the precise localization is only obtainable from the *coronal* set [Figure 4.18]. In this instance, the patient had a superior left quadrantanopia and a partial inferior quadrantic defect. By themselves, these findings would tell us that the lesion

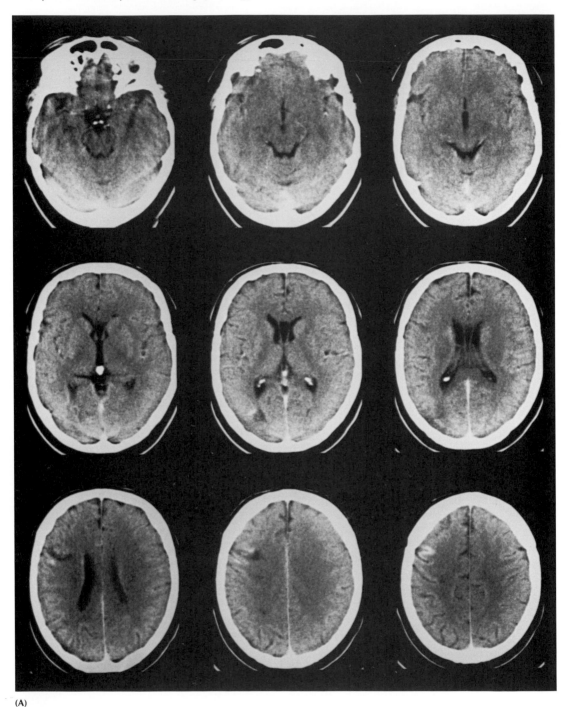

(A)

FIGURE 4.11. CT (A) of a 41-year-old man with a nonfluent aphasia and a remarkably preserved ability to repeat sentences. The condition conforms to the category of transcortical motor aphasia. Note the distinction between this profile and that of mutism with akinesia, in which no intent to communicate is detectable and in which true linguistic errors are rare.

Corresponding template (B) with charted lesion involving the left dorsolateral frontal lobe (en-

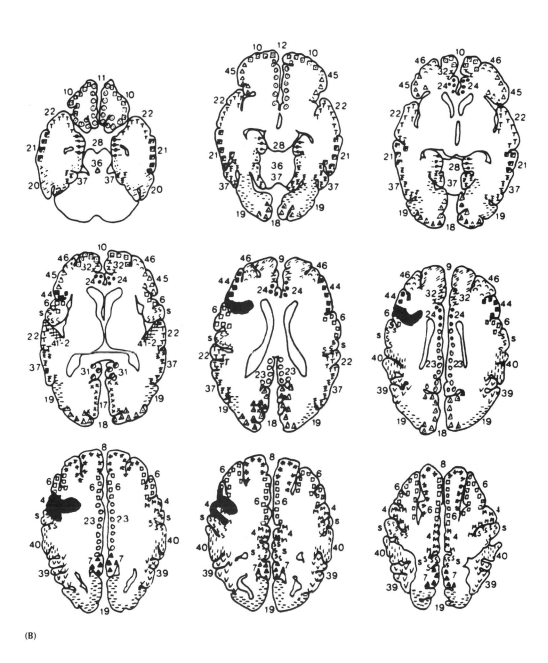

(B)

compassing the pre-motor area immediately above the frontal operculum, that is, area 6 above area 44. The lesion barely involves the superior-most portion of areas 44 and 45. It extends to the motor cortex just posterior to these areas. The white matter immediately underneath is involved, but the deep white matter closer to the wall of the ventricle is spared.

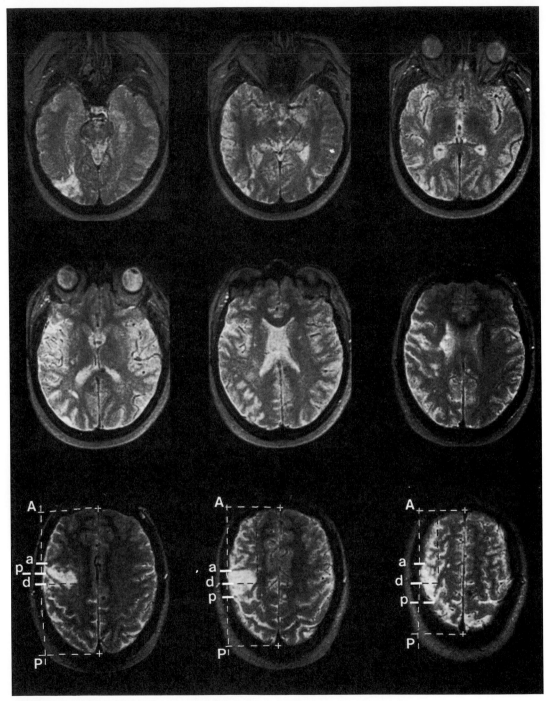

(A)

FIGURE 4.12. (A) MR (T$_2$ weighted image) of the patient whose CT is shown in Figure 4.11.

(B) Careful search for the best-fitting template system reveals that none of the available sets really fit the scan. Even our most horizontal set still does not fit the incidence. Compare the third cut on the right in (A), with the second and third cuts on the template. The MR cut barely involves the lowest portion of the frontal lobe and already cuts posteriorly through the splenium of the corpus

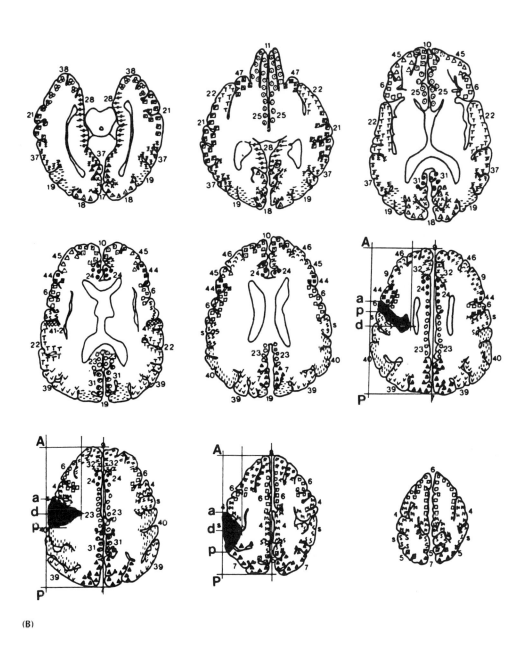

(B)

callosum. Cuts 2 and 3 in the template set fit, respectively, the anterior portion (cut 2) and the posterior portion (cut 3) of the MR cut. Using this set, with strict ''blind'' x/y plotting approach, the lesion would fall mainly in the parietal lobe.

The first (lowest) MR cut also shows an infarct in the lateral occipital region (which is also seen in the fifth cut of the CT in Figure 4.11).

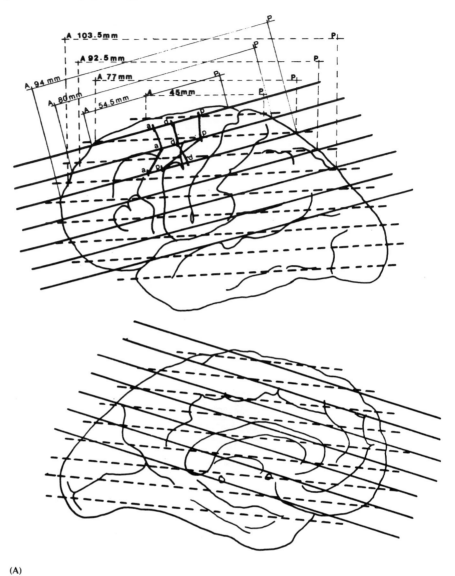

(A)

FIGURE 4.13. There is a cumbersome means to plot lesions seen in "nonconforming" scans such as the one in Figure 4.12A, which was obtained with a negative tilt. Shown here (A) are lateral and mesial brain diagrams with lines corresponding to tem-plate cuts (dotted line) and to MR cuts (solid line). The plotting requires the following steps:

1. X/Y plot transfer of the limits of the lesion to the lateral brain.

2. Joining of the points corresponding to the

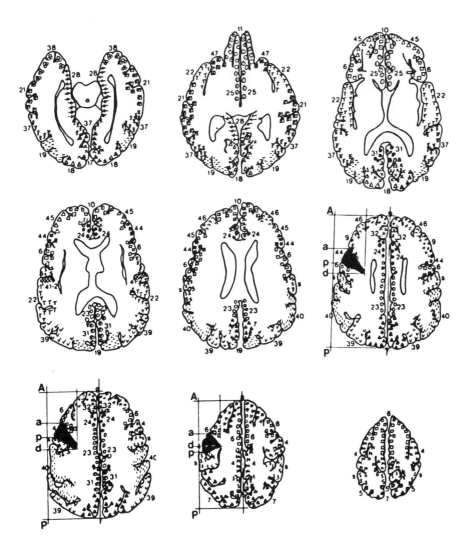

(B)

anterior (a), posterior (p), and deep (d) limits of the lesion, at each level.

3. Determination of the points at which the line circumscribing the limits of the lesion crosses the dotted line corresponding to the template cuts.

4. Transfer of these points to the template system (B). As expected, this plotting reveals the lesion to be in the same location indicated by CT (Figure 4.10).

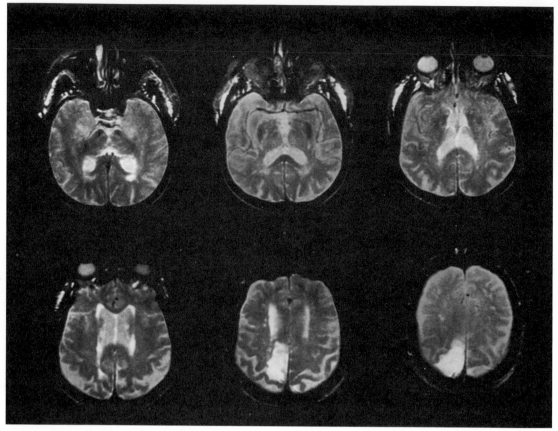

(A)

FIGURE 4.14. MR of an 81-year-old, right-handed man who suddenly developed a right-sided motor deficit. He had severe weakness in his leg and arm, but none in the hand or face.

(A) The T_2 weighted MR obtained five days after onset showed an area of bright signal in the left hemisphere. (B and C) After appropriate plotting using the method described in Figure 4.13, it was evident that the lesion was in the mesial motor cortex and underlying white matter with extension into the mesial portion of the cingulate gyrus. (See also Figures 4.15 and 4.20).

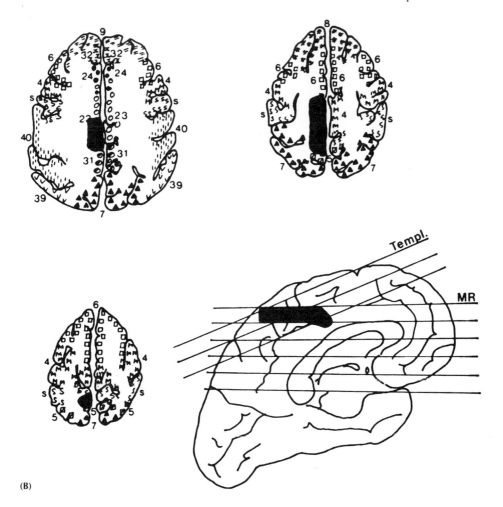

(B)

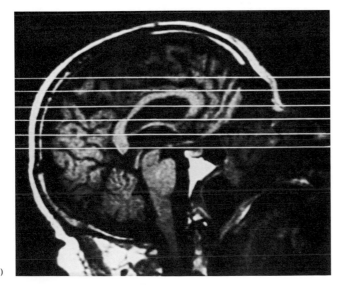

(C)

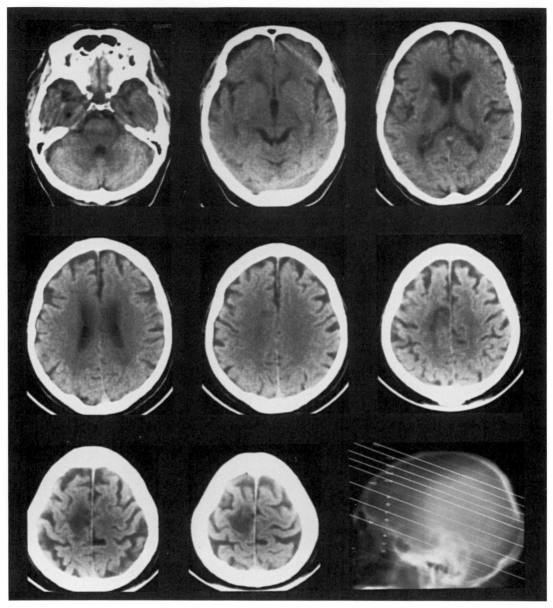

(A)

FIGURE 4.15. Chronic CT (A) and corresponding templates (B) of the patient seen in Figure 4.14, obtained with a more standard angulation. It shows both the recent infarct in the mesial motor cortex, and an old lacune in the caudate nucleus.

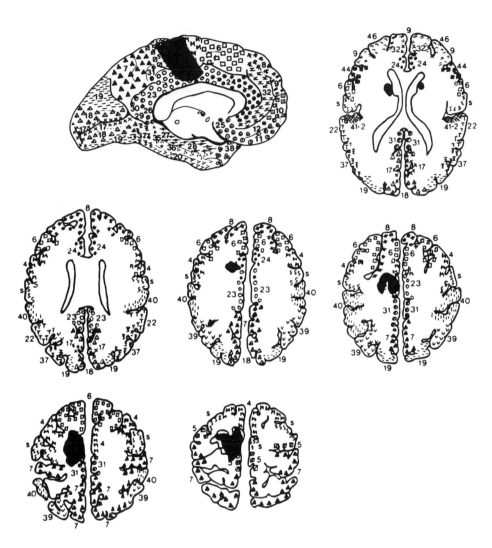

(B)

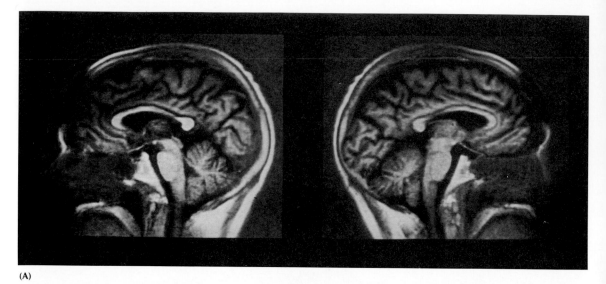

(A)

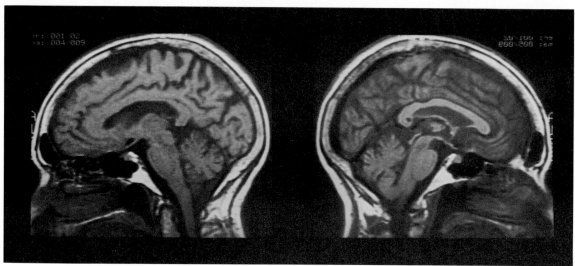

(B)

FIGURE 4.16. MR (T$_1$ weighted) sagittal cuts of the left and right hemispheres in two different subjects. Inspection of the mesial surface of the occipital lobes shows that the course taken by the calcarine fissure is different in subjects (A) and (B). In fact, even in the same subject, the left and right calcarine fissures may assume a different course.

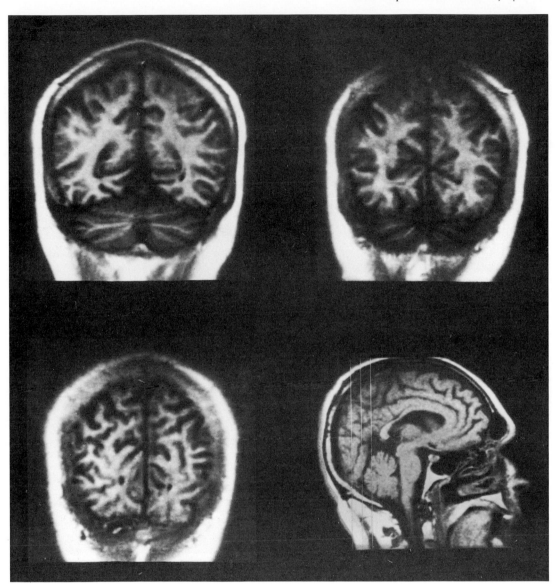

FIGURE 4.17. MR (T$_1$ weighted) coronal cuts of the occipital lobe. The insert on the right-hand side corner shows a midsagittal cut with markings corresponding to the three cuts above. The calcarine fissure, which is clearly seen in the midsagittal cut, can easily be followed in three coronal cuts. Cut number 2 shows the typical image of two letter V's placed sideways (><). The Vs correspond to the juncture of the calcarine and the parieto-occipital sulcus.

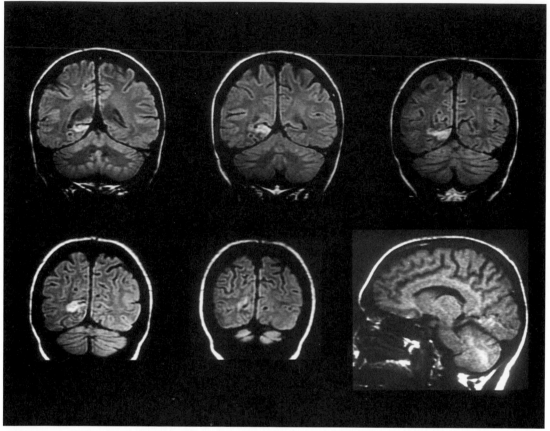

(A)

FIGURE 4.18. MR of a subject with a right occipital infarct. In (A), the infarct is clearly seen in the infracalcarine region, in both coronal and midsagittal cuts. In (B), however, the calcarine fissure cannot be identified. From this image, the infarct appears to be in the infracalcarine region because it is only seen in the second cut, but that assumption cannot be verified. It is not possible to say if the lesion involves both banks of the calcarine sulcus, a pattern that would cause a hemianopia, or if it damages only the inferior calcarine bank, a pattern that should cause only a superior quadrantanopia. In this instance, the patient had a complete left superior quadrantanopia and a par-

was predominantly infracalcarine. But the lesion also involved part of the superior lip of the calcarine region striate cortex.

The transverse cuts alone might have suggested the possibility of an infracalcarine lesion because the area of abnormal signal was only seen in the lower cut. But the study of the coronal cut is the one that shows unequivocally that the lesion is infracalcarine. However, it does not allow us to determine whether it involves both lips of the calcarine sulcus. Figure 4.19 shows another example of a patient

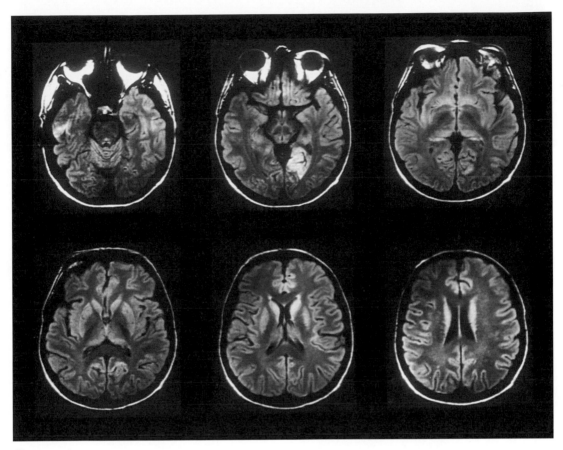

(B)

tial defect in the lower quadrant, indicating that the lesion involved both the inferior bank and part of the superior bank of the calcarine region.

It is interesting to compare this patient with the one discussed in Figure 2.5. Unlike that achromatopsic individual, this patient has *both* normal form vision and normal color vision in the remainder of

the left, unaffected visual field. This indicates that the lesion, as the coronal cut demonstrates, destroys primary visual cortex in the infracalcarine region, but does not extend enough into infracalcarine association cortices so as to impinge on the "color dedicated" visual association cortices.

with a visual field defect. In this case, the patient had a right homonymous hemianopia. From the analysis of these two MRs, however, it would not be possible to predict that a difference existed in the visual fields of these two patients.

The advantage of having a midsagittal image to achieve an easy identification of the calcarine fissure is obvious. However, such a cut may be essential for other reasons. Figure 3.10 shows an example of the posterior coronal cuts of a patient with Pick's disease. It is

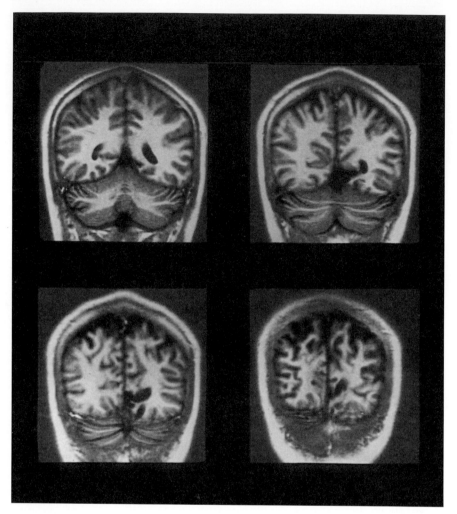

FIGURE 4.19. MR (T$_1$ weighted images) of a 29-year-old, right-handed man who had sustained a left occipital infarct three weeks earlier. The lesion caused a dense right homonymous hemianopia. No other abnormalities could be detected.

The MR images show an area of abnormally low signal in the left infracalcarine and calcarine region. In this case, however, it is impossible to verify the full extent of calcarine region involvement (as opposed to the previous example in Figure 4.18), although the lesion must extend to the upper bank of the calcarine region.

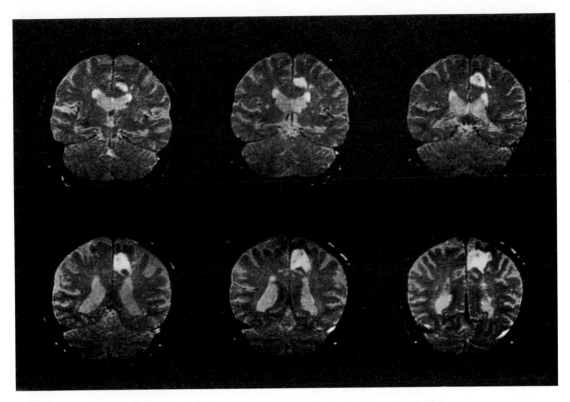

FIGURE 4.20. Coronal T₂ weighted MR cuts of the patient seen in Figure 4.14. This image shows that the abnormal area of bright signal involves part of the cingulate gyrus, the mesial motor cortex, and white matter underlying both.

well-known that this particular type of degenerative dementia mostly affects the anterior frontal and temporal lobes, resulting in marked "lobar" atrophy. In this example, however, the images seem to suggest that the atrophy extends all the way into the occipital lobe. On the other hand, the midsagittal cut of a pilot scan reveals that these cuts were not obtained at a 90 degree angle in relation to the inferior orbitomeatal line, and that, in fact, the most-posterior cuts in the scan are merely cutting through the most-posterior regions of the frontal lobe and the parietal lobe's anterior region.

In the case of the patient with right hemiparesis sparing the hand and face, shown in Figure 4.14, the inspection of the coronal cuts would have led to the correct interpretation of the lesion. It is evident that the infarct is in the mesial frontoparietal region and it damages the mesial aspect of the motor cortex, as well as part of the posterior cingulate gyrus [Figure 4.20].

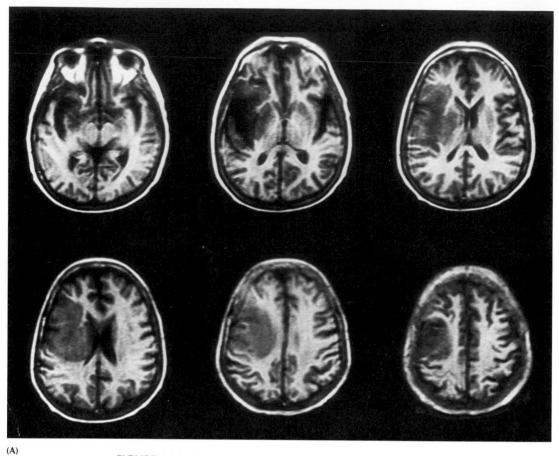

(A)

FIGURE 4.21. Acute T₁ weighted MR (A) and corresponding templates (B) of a 65-year-old woman who developed global aphasia. These T₁ weighted, transverse images show a large area of low signal in the left frontal operculum, the insula, and the basal ganglia. The abnormal area extends posteriorly into the anterior parietal regions and seems to extend into anterior portions of the temporal lobe, in cut 3. As can be seen in Figure 4.22, that is not so.

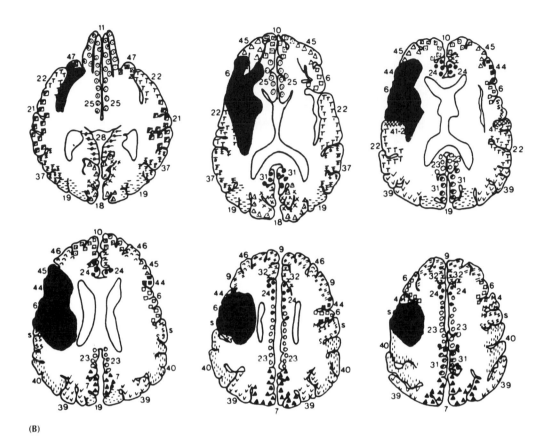

(B)

Coronal cuts are also far superior for detailed analysis of the temporal structures. Most anatomical details are readily recognizable in coronal views, especially in MR images of the T_1 weighted variety. Not only are the different gyri clearly identifiable, but not infrequently, the transverse gyri of Heshl can be well-visualized, virtually subdividing the superior temporal gyrus in anterior and posterior sections. The parahippocampal gyrus, the hippocampal formation proper, and the amygdala can be visualized also [see Figures 3.18–20]. Coronal cuts are also crucial to decide on the extension of lesions across lobar boundaries, for example, the extension of a frontal lesion into the superior temporal region, or the extension of posterior temporal lesions into the parietal lobe located immediately above. Figures 4.21 and 4.22 provide illustrative examples.

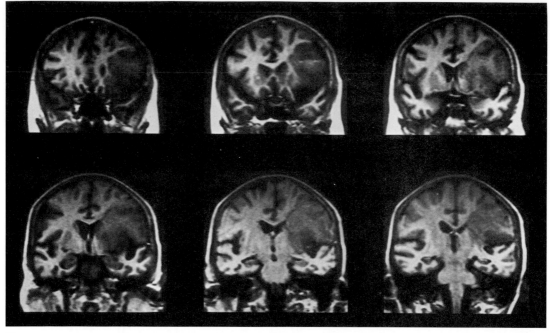

(A)

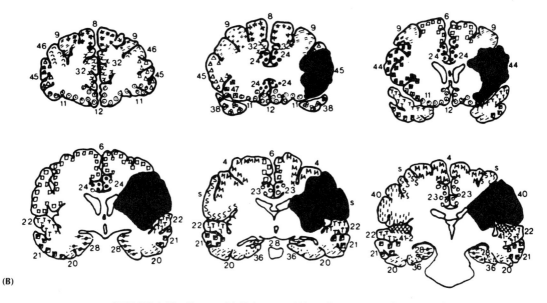

(B)

FIGURE 4.22. Coronal MR images (A) and corresponding template (B) of the same patient of Figure 4.21. These T$_1$ weighted images were obtained the same day as the transverse cuts. Careful inspection of these images shows that the left temporal lobe is not only spared in its posterior portion, as can be surmised from the transverse cuts, but is intact even anteriorly. The damage is circumscribed to the frontal and parietal lobes.

This is one of several patterns of left hemisphere damage that can cause global aphasia. It resembles the pattern described in Figure 2.19 and differs from those described in Figures 2.17 and 2.18.

180

References

Braak H: The pigment architecture of the human temporal lobe. *Anatomy of Embryology,* **154:**213–240, 1978.

Brodmann K: *Vergleichende Lokalisationlehre der Grosshirnrinde.* Leipzig, J. A. Barth, 1909.

Damasio H: A computed tomographic guide to the identification of cerebral vascular territories. *Archives of Neurology* **40:**138–142, 1983.

Damasio H: Vascular territories defined by computerized tomography. In Wood JH (ed.): *Cerebral Blood Flow: Physiologic and Clinical Aspects,* pp. 324–332. New York, McGraw-Hill, 1987.

DeArmond SJ, Fusco MM, Dewey MM: *Structure of the Human Brain, A Photographic Atlas.* New York, Oxford University Press, 1976.

Gado M, Hanaway J, Frank R: Functional anatomy of the cerebral cortex by computed tomography. *Journal of Computerized Axial Tomography* **3:**1–19, 1979.

Graff-Radford NR, Damasio H, Yamada T, Eslinger PJ, Damasio A: Nonhemorrhagic thalamic infarction. *Brain* **108:**485–516, 1985.

Hanaway J, Scott WR, Strother CM. *Atlas of the Human Brain and the Orbit for Computed Tomography.* St. Louis, MO, Warren H. Green Inc., 1977.

Lazorthes G, Gouaze A, Salamon G: *Vascularisation et circulation de l'encephale.* Paris, Masson, 1976.

Matsui T, Hirano A: *An Atlas of the Human Brain for Computerized Tomography.* Tokyo, Igaku-Shoin Ltd, 1978.

Palacios E, Fine M, Henghton VM: *Multiplanar Anatomy of the Head and Neck: For Computed Tomography.* New York, John Wiley & Sons, 1980.

Salamon G, Huang YP: *Radiologic Anatomy of the Brain.* Berlin, Springer Verlag, 1976.

Sarkissow SA, Filimonoft IN, Konowa EP, et al.: *Atlas of the Cytoarchitectonics of the Human Cerebral Cortex.* Moscow, Medgiz, 1955.

Schnitzlein H, Murtagh F: *Imaging Anatomy of the Head and Spine.* Baltimore, MD, Urban and Schwarzenberg, 1985.

Talairach J, Szikla G: *Atlas d'anatomie stéréotaxique du télencéphale.* Paris, Masson et Cie, 1967.

Waddington MM: *Atlas of Cerebral Angiography With Anatomic Correlation.* Boston, Little Brown & Co., 1974.

APPENDIX

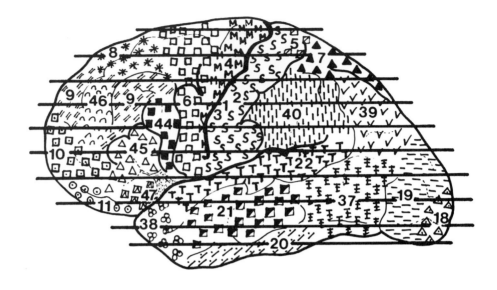

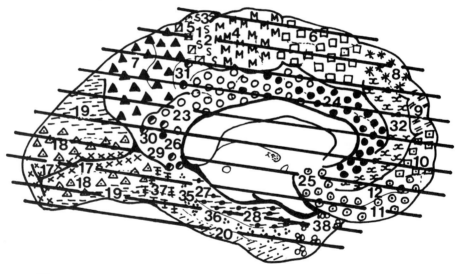

(A)

FIGURE A.1.

FIGURES A.1–A.6. Six different sets of templates with cytoarchitectonic markings. The first set corresponds to the most horizontal incidence (parallel to the inferior orbitomeatal line). The last corresponds to cuts obtained at a 90 degree angle to this same line. Other sets correspond to intermediate incidences. The template sets are matched with the mesial and lateral views of a left hemisphere drawing, onto which lines corresponding to the level of incidence and orientation of the template set have been marked.

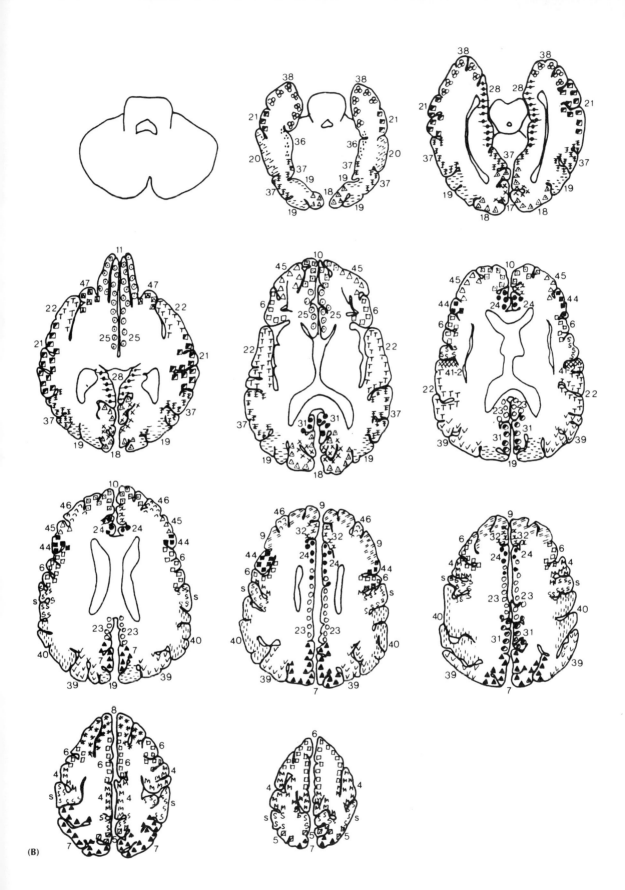

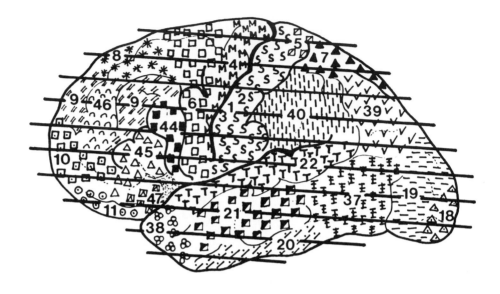

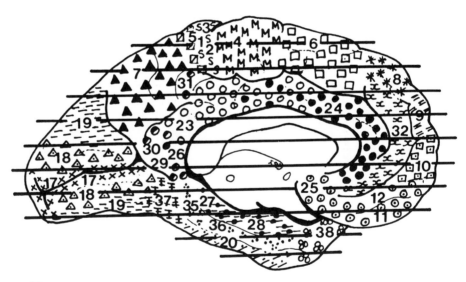

(A)

FIGURE A.2.

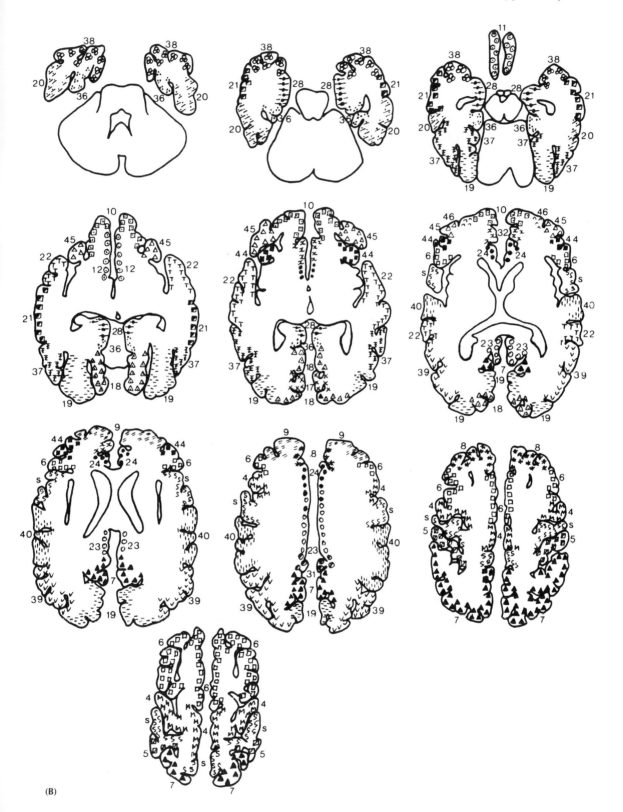

(B)

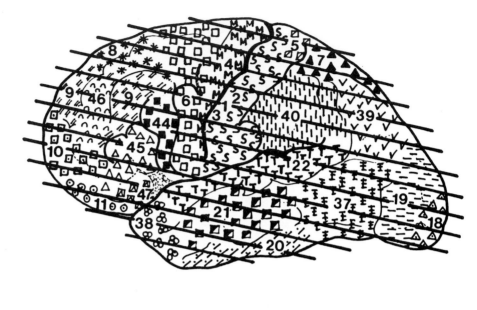

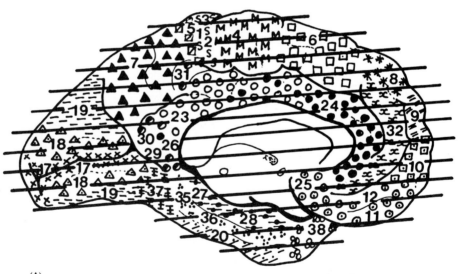

(A)

FIGURE A.3.

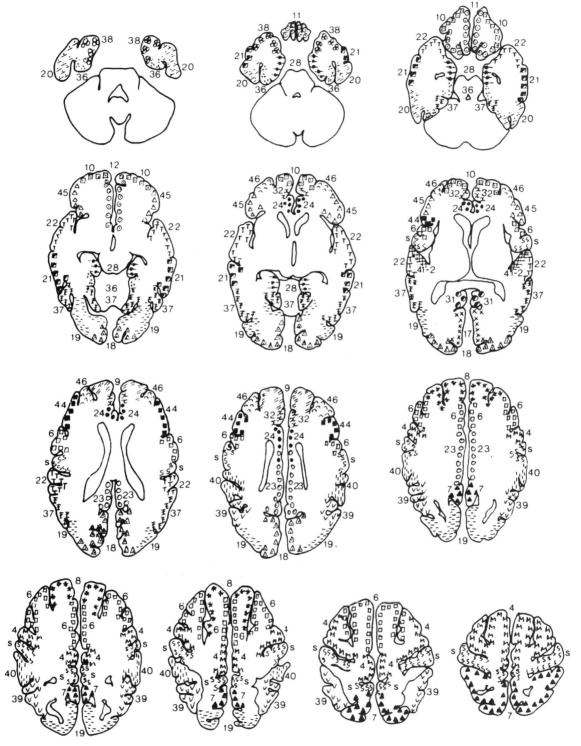

(B)

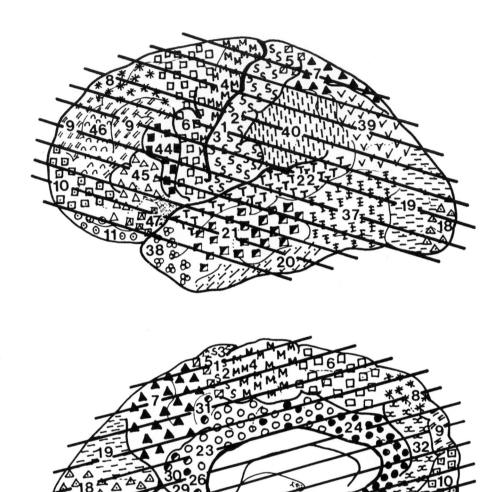

(A)

FIGURE A.4.

190

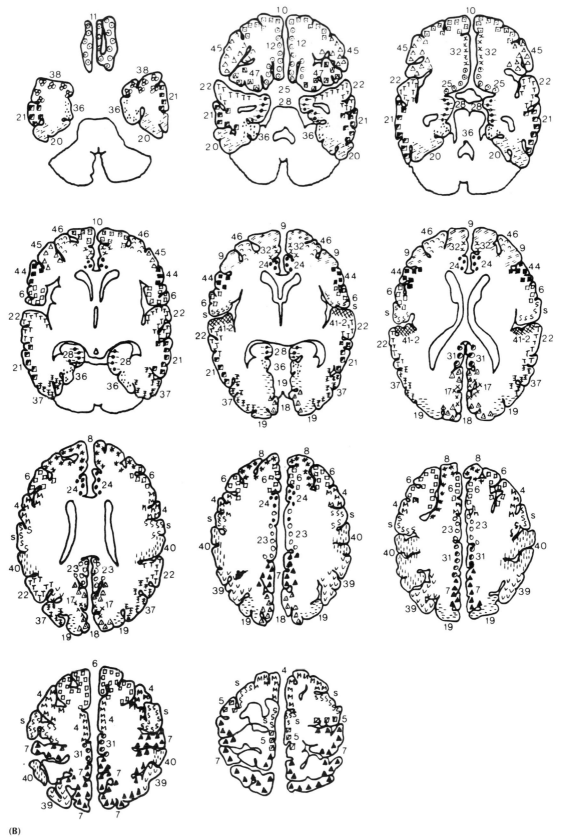

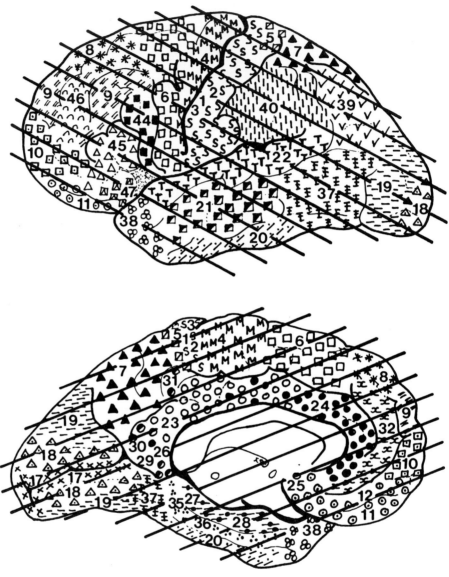

(A)

FIGURE A.5.

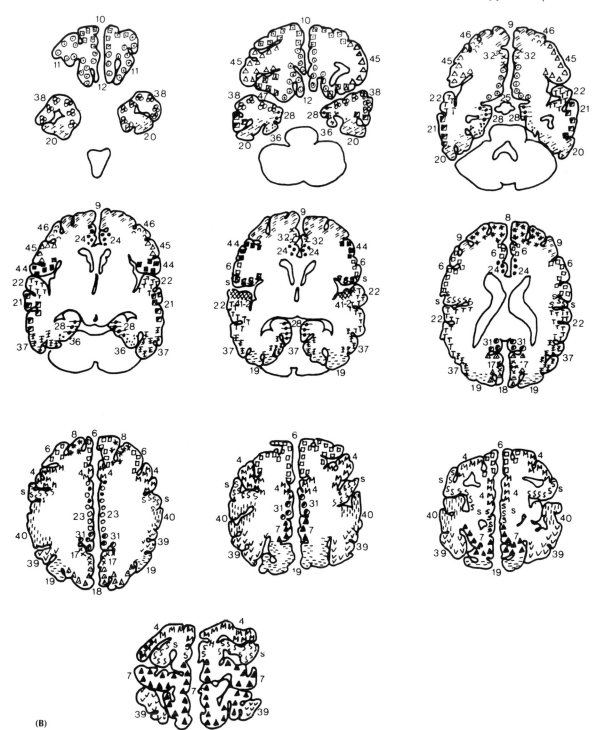

(B)

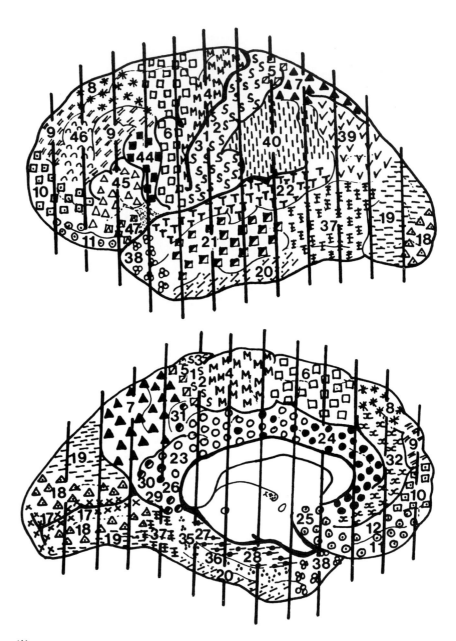

(A)

FIGURE A.6.

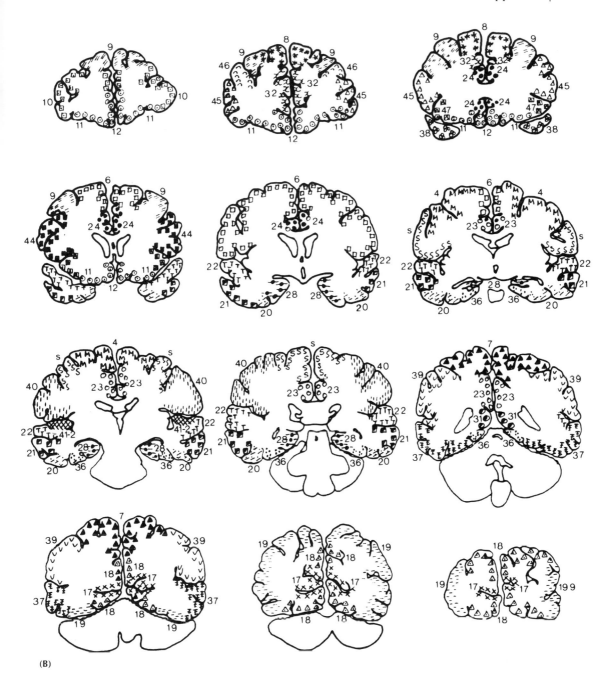

(B)

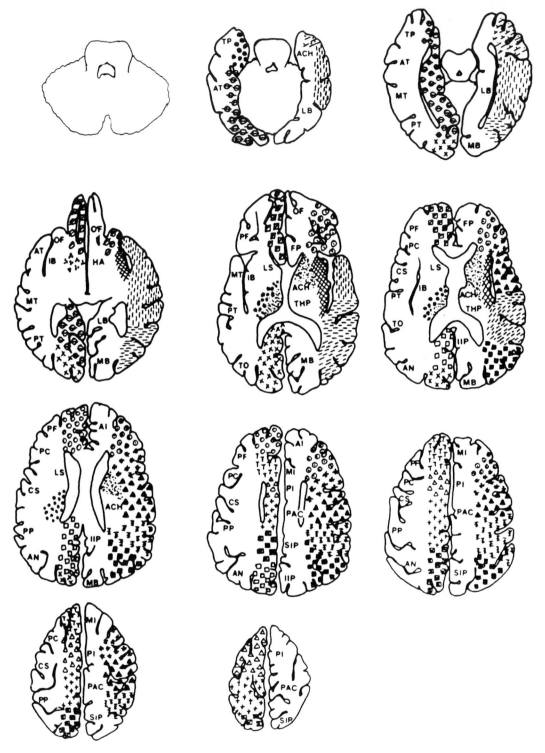

FIGURE A.7.

FIGURES A.7–A.11. Same set of templates as in Figures A.1–A.6 for *transverse* cuts, with markings corresponding to the distribution of the branches of (a) the middle cerebral artery within the left hemisphere, and (b) the anterior and posterior ce-

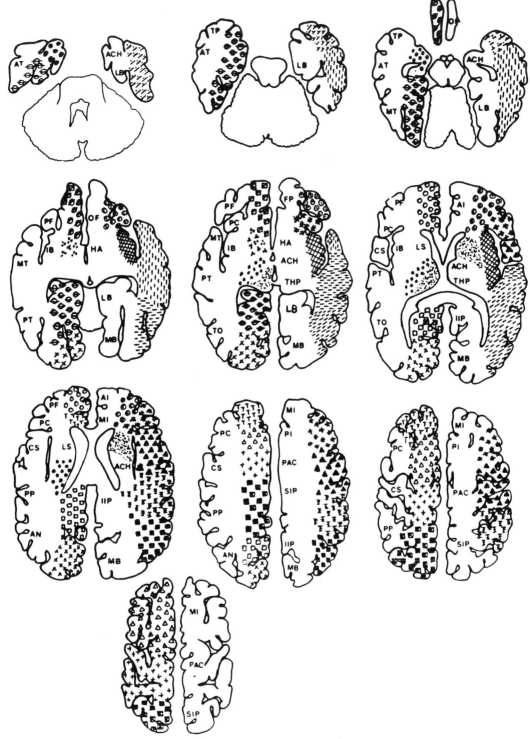

FIGURE A.8.

rebral arteries within the right hemisphere. (Modified from H. Damasio, in Wood
J (ed): *Cerebral Blood Flow: Physiologic and Clinical Aspects*, pp 324–332. New
York, McGraw-Hill, 1987).

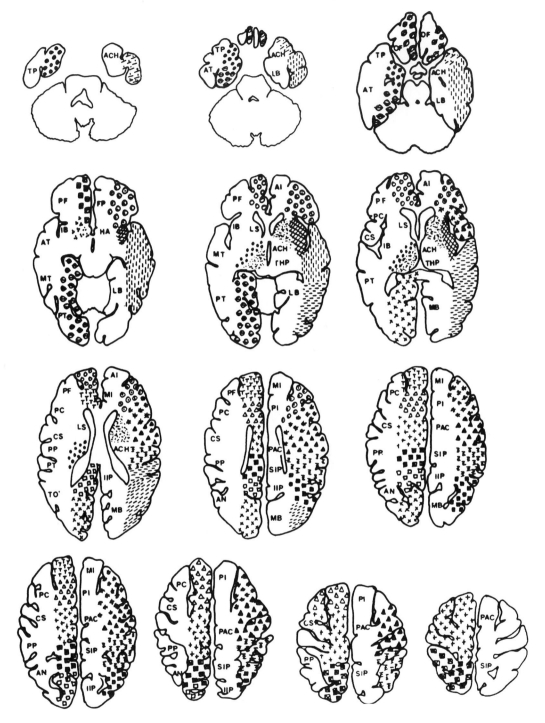

FIGURE A.9.

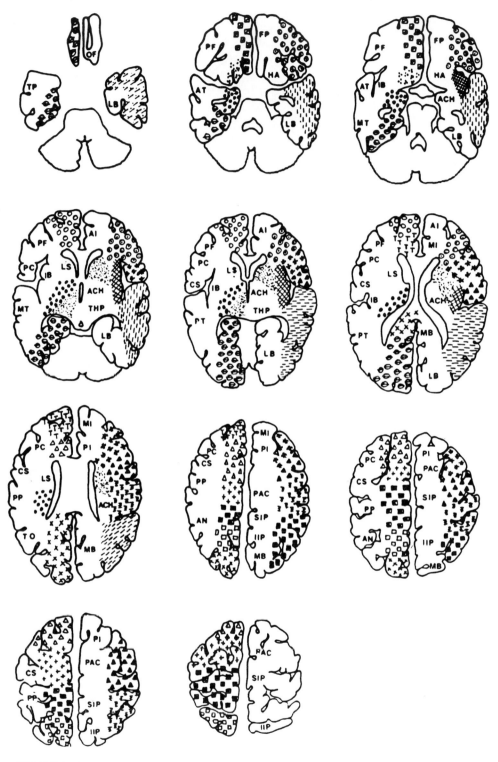

FIGURE A.10.

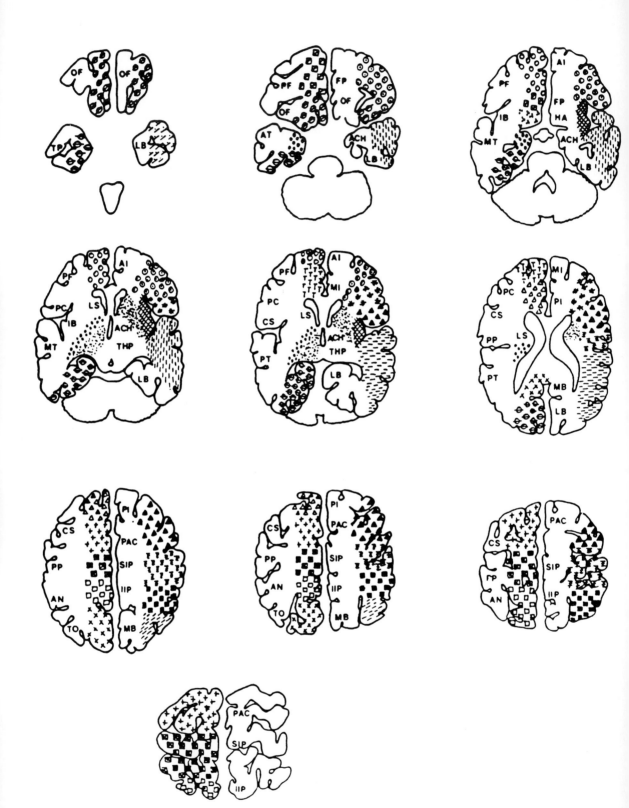

FIGURE A.11.

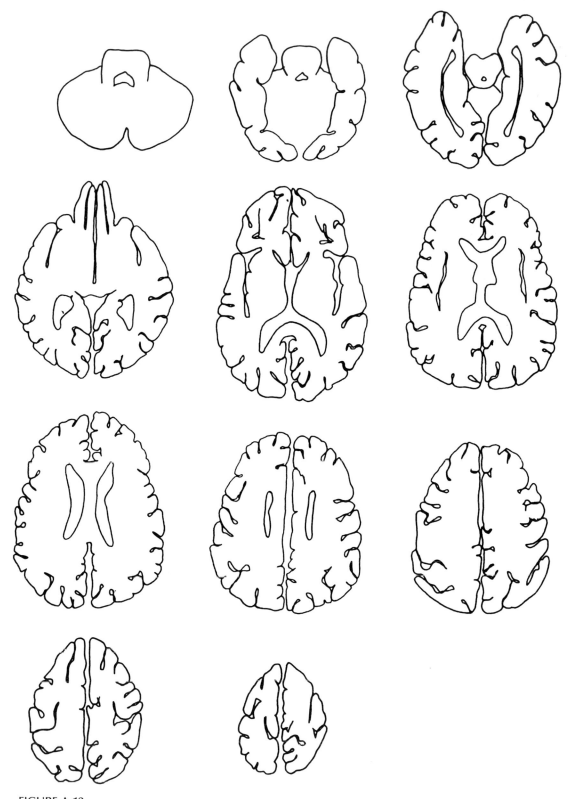

FIGURE A.12.

FIGURES A.12–A.17. Same sets of six templates seen in Figures A.1B through A.6B, but without cytoarchitectonic markings. These are used to chart the CT/MR lesions for research purposes.

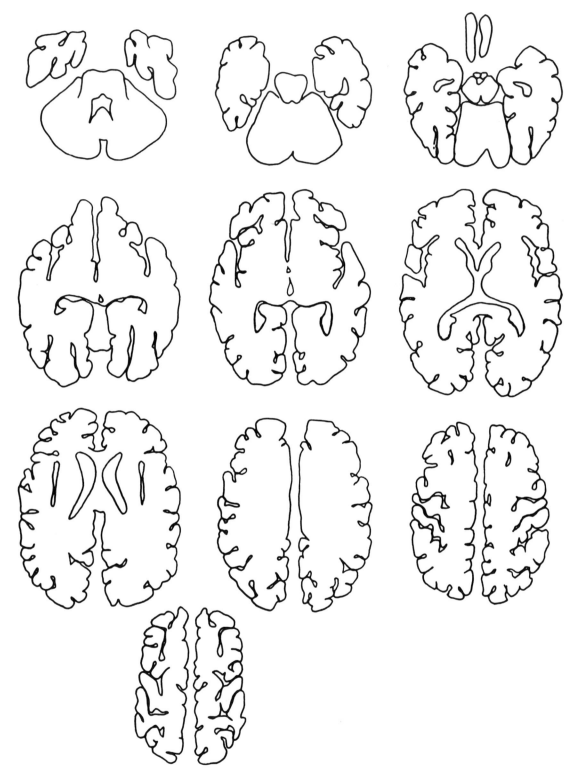

FIGURE A.13.

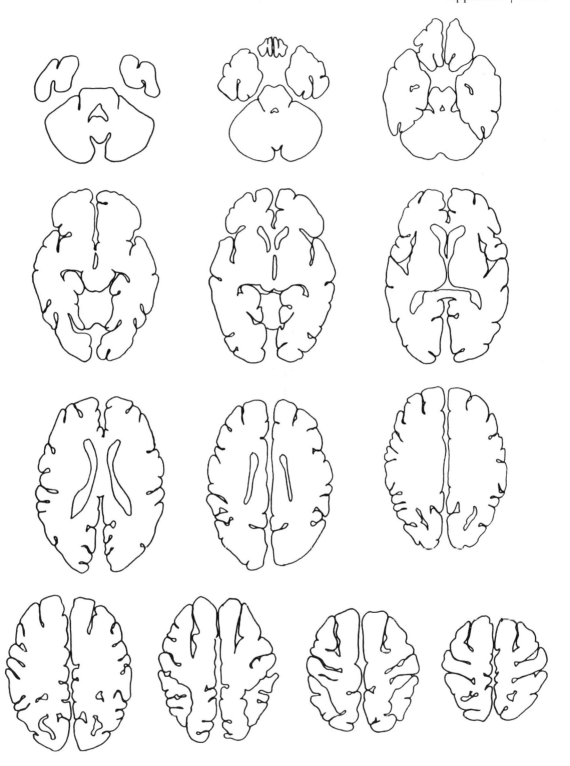

FIGURE A.14.

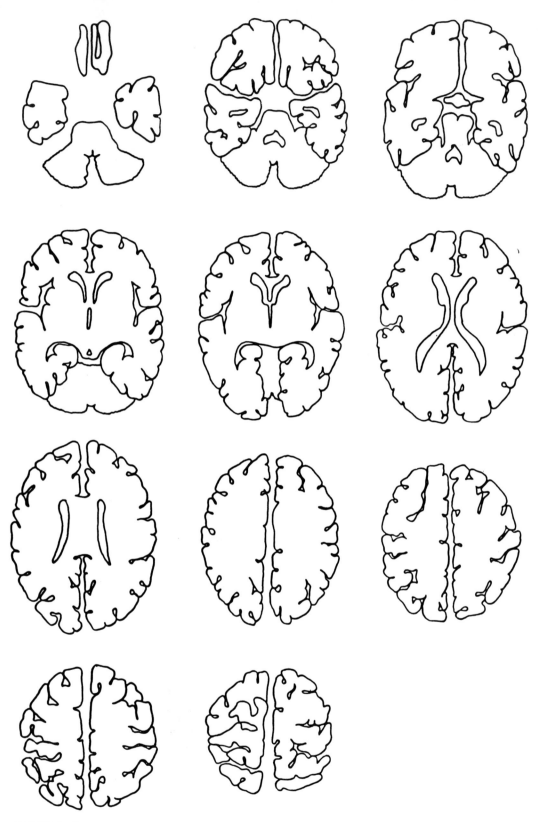

FIGURE A.15.

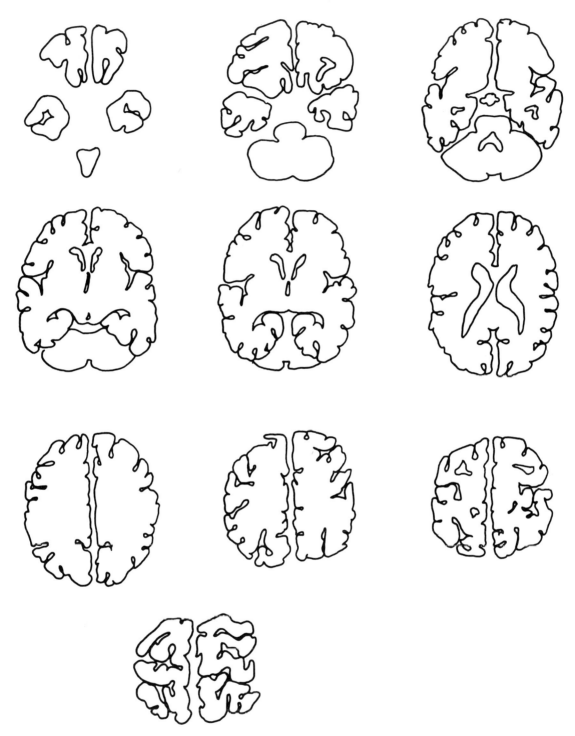

FIGURE A.16.

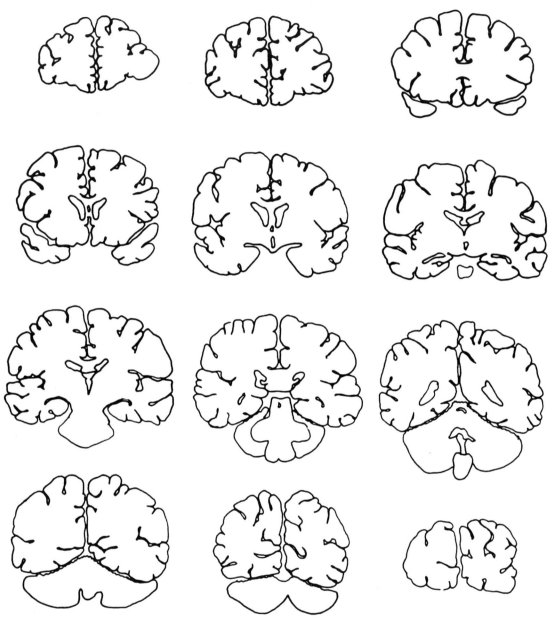

FIGURE A.17.

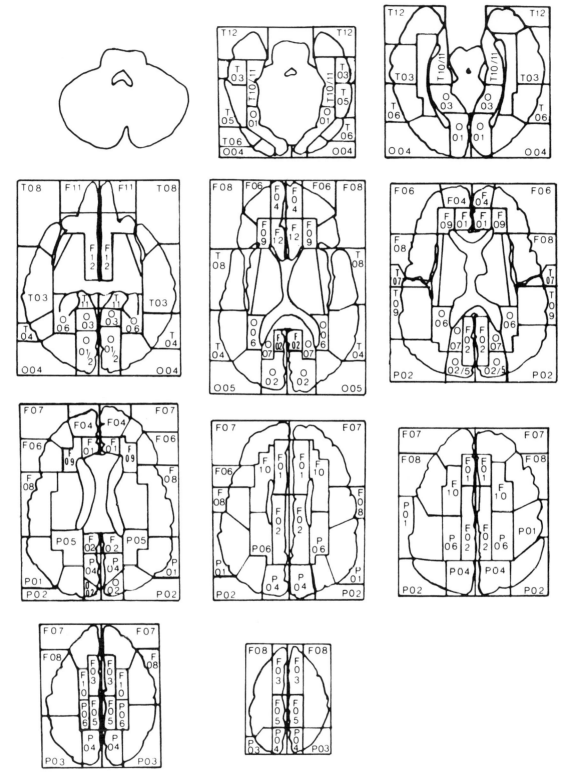

FIGURE A.18.

FIGURES A.18–A.23. Same sets of six templates with cells of anatomical areas of interest, keyed to research interests of our laboratory (see Table A.1 for the code of the cells).

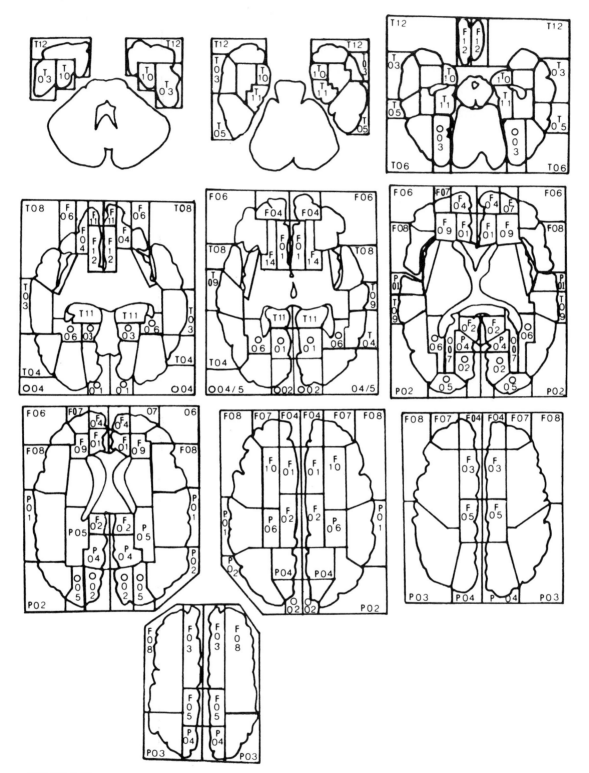

FIGURE A.19.

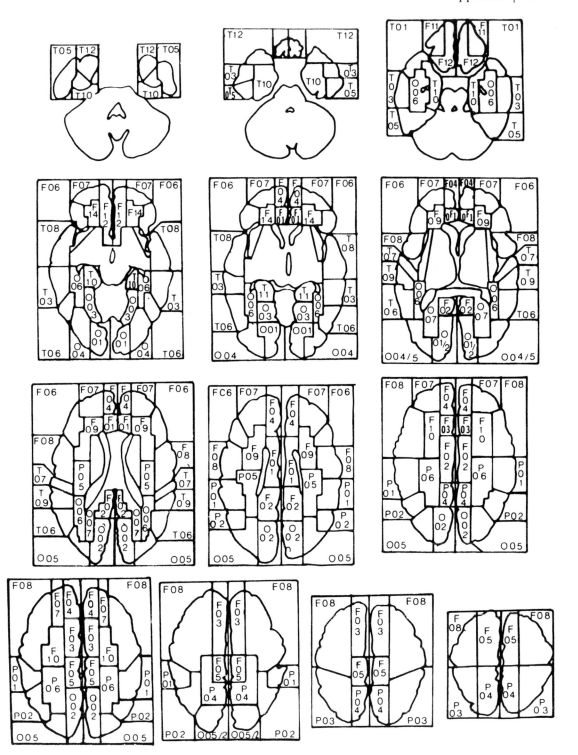

FIGURE A.20.

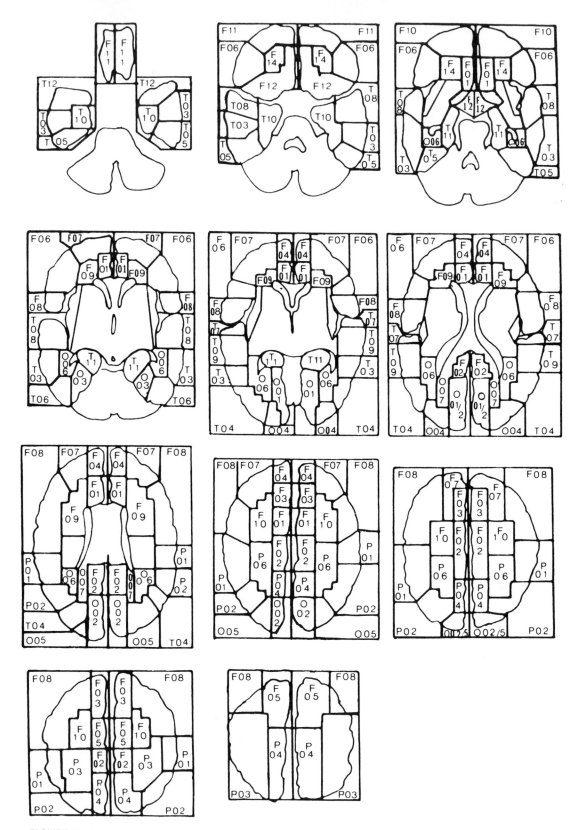

FIGURE A.21.

210

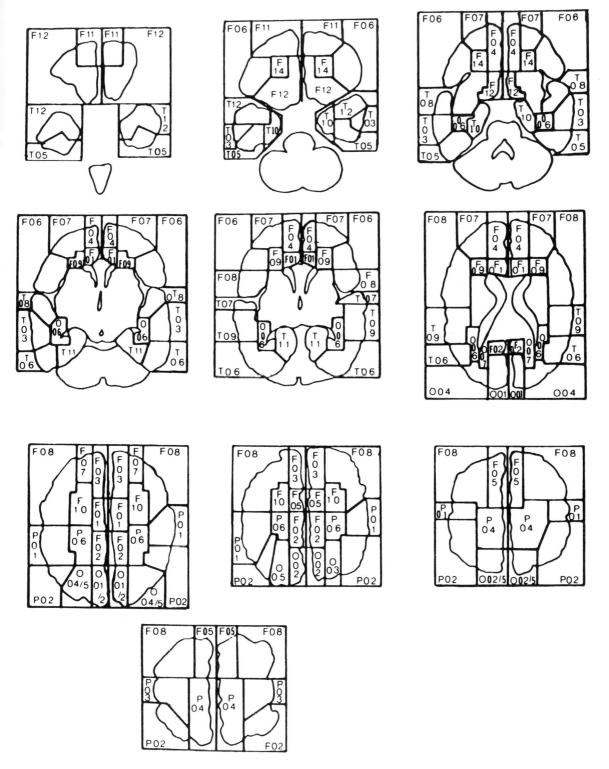

FIGURE A.22.

211

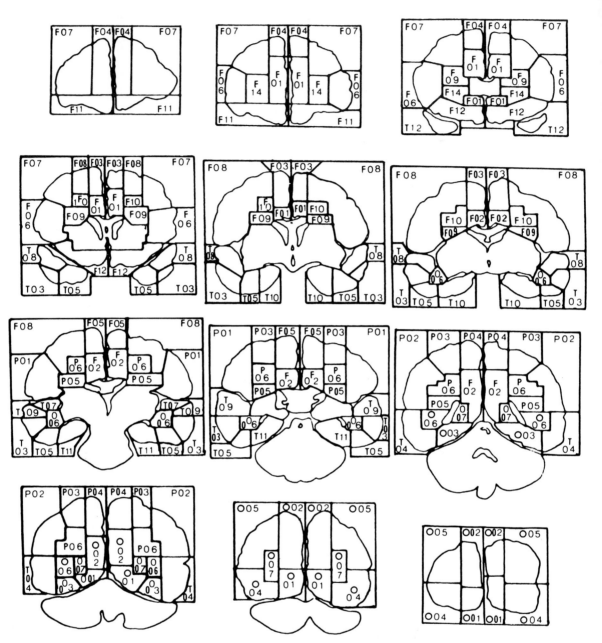

FIGURE A.23.

212

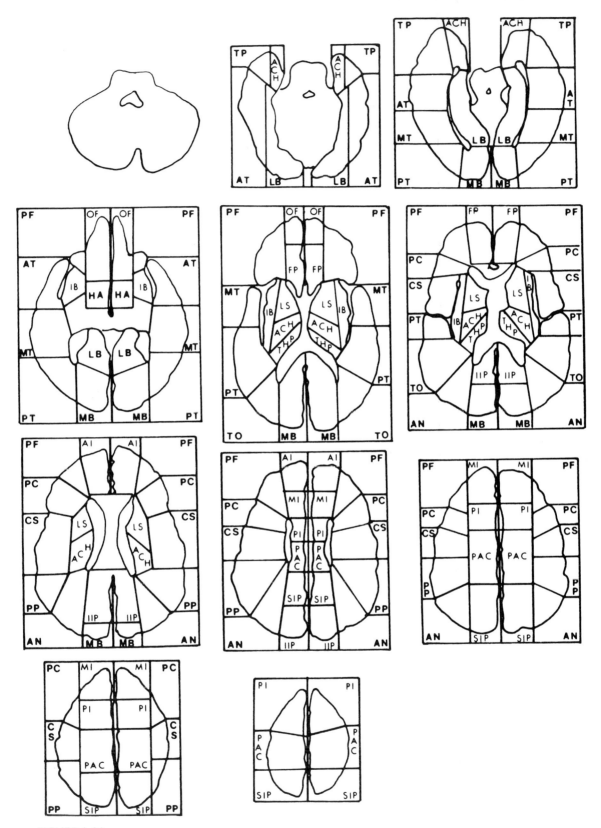

FIGURE A.24.

FIGURES A.24–A.28. Same sets of five transverse templates with cells of *vascular territories* (see Table A.2 for the code of the cells).

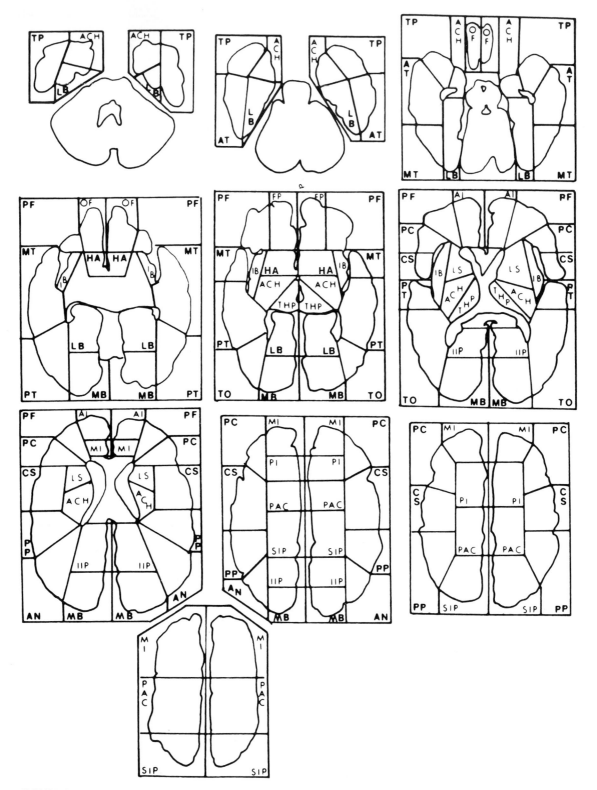

FIGURE A.25.

214

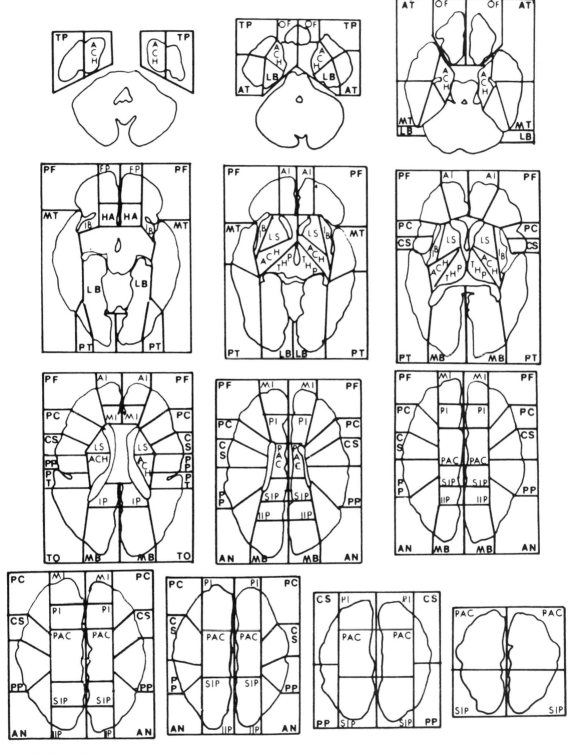

FIGURE A.26.

215

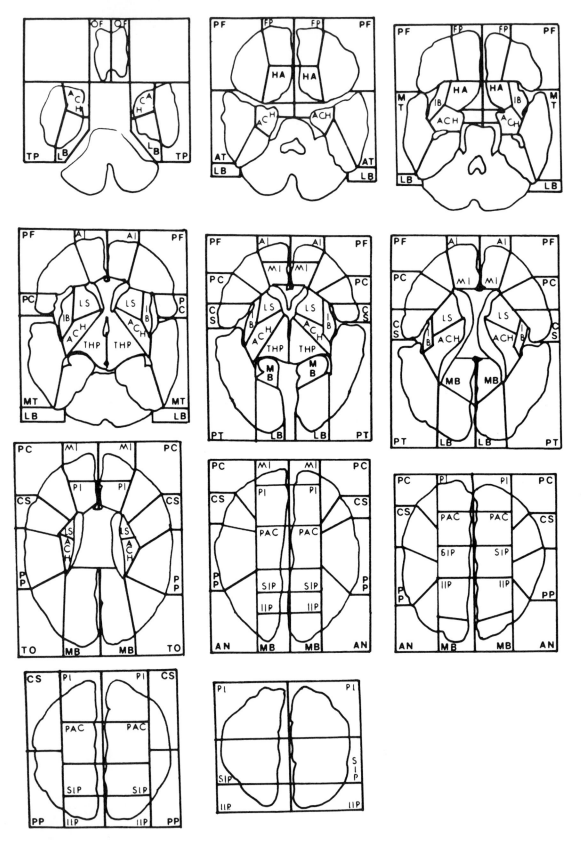

FIGURE A.27.

216

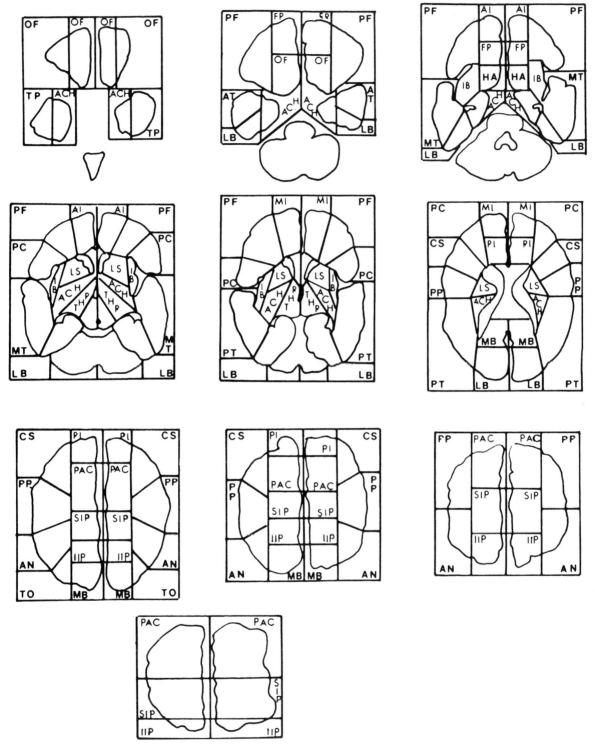

FIGURE A.28.

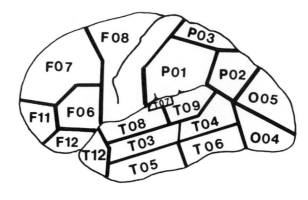

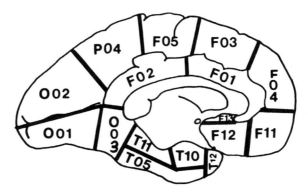

FIGURE A.29. Drawing of the lateral and mesial brian with markings of anatomical areas of interest, used in Figures A.19 through A.24, projected onto the outer surfaces of the brain.

Table A.1. Key to the code used in the identification of anatomical areas of interest

FRONTAL LOBE

Mesial Aspect

F01	Cingulate Gyrus	anterior (24)
F02		posterior (23, 31)
F03	Supplementary Motor Area (6)	
F04	Prefrontal Region (8, 9, 10)	
F05	Rolandic Region (4, 3, 1, 2)	

Lateral Aspect

F06	Frontal Operculum (44, 45)	
F07	Pre-frontal Region (8, 9, 46)	
F08	Pre-motor Region (6)	
	Rolandic Region (4, 3, 1, 2)	
F09	Paraventricular	
F10	Supraventricular Area	

Orbital Aspect

F11	Anterior (10)
F12	Posterior (11, 12, 13, 47)
F13	Basal Forebrain
F14	Subventricular Area

TEMPORAL LOBE

Lateral/Superior Aspect

T03	Middle Temp. Gyrus	anterior (21)
T04		posterior (37)
T05	Inferior Temp. Gyrus	anterior (20)
T06		posterior (37)
T07	Auditory Region (41, 42)	
T08	Anterior to Auditory Region (22)	
T09	Posterior to Auditory Region (22)	

Mesial Aspect

T10	Anterior (Amygdala, 28, 36)
T11	Posterior (Hippocampus, 28, 36)
T12	*Polar Area (38)*

PARIETAL LOBE

Inferior Parietal Lobule

P01	Supramarginal Gyrus (40)
P02	Angular Gyrus (39)

Superior Parietal Lobule

P03	Lateral (7, 5)
P04	Mesial (7, 5)
P05	Paraventricular Area
P06	Supraventricular Area

OCCIPITAL LOBE

Mesial Aspect

001	Infracalcarine (18, 19)
002	Supracalcarine (18, 19)
003	Temporo-occipital Junction (37, 36)

Lateral Aspect

004	Inferior (18, 19)
005	Superior (18, 19)
006	Paraventricular Area
007	Forceps major

INSULA

I01	Anterior
I02	Posterior

CENTRAL GRAY AND ADJOINING WHITE MATTER

Basal Ganglia

BG1	Caudate Nucleus	Head
BG2		Body
BG3	Lenticular Nucleus	Putamen
BG4		Pallidum

Thalamus

TH1	Anterior
TH2	Posterior
TH3	Lateral
TH4	Mesial

Internal capsule

IC1	Anterior Limb
IC2	Posterior Limb
IC3	Genu
HYT	*Hypothalamus*

CORPUS CALLOSUM

C01	Genu
C02	Body
C03	Splenium

Table A.2. Key to the code used in the definition of vascular territories

ANTERIOR CEREBRAL ARTERY

Orbito-frontal	OF	AC0
Fronto-polar	FP	
Anterior Internal Frontal	AI	
Middle Internal Frontal	MI	AC1
Posterior Internal Frontal	PI	
Paracentral	PAC	AC2
Superior Internal Parietal	SIP	AC3
Inferior Internal Parietal	IIP	
Heubner's Artery	HA	AC4
Callosal Arteries		AC5

POSTERIOR CEREBRAL ARTERY

Lateral Branch	LB	PC1
Medial Branch	MB	PC2
Thalamoperforating	THP	PC3

ANTERIOR CHOROIDAL   ACH   ACH

MIDDLE CEREBRAL ARTERY

Orbito-Frontal	OF	MC1
Pre-frontal	PF	
Pre-central	PC	MC2
Central	CS	
Posterior Parietal	PP	MC3
Angular	AN	
Temporo-occipital	TO	
Temporo-polar	TP	MC4
Anterior Temporal	AT	
Middle Temporal	MT	MC5
Posterior Temporal	PT	
Lenticulo-striate	LS	MC6
Insular Branches	IB	MC7

Table A.3. Key to the symbols used for cytoarchitectonic areas.

Symbol	Brodmann designation	Neuroanatomical designations
M	area 4	precentral gyrus; primary motor cortex
■	area 44	pars opercularis ⎱
△	area 45	pars triangularis ⎬ frontal operculum; on the left, the combination of 44 and 45 = Broca area
⊠	area 47	pars orbitalis ⎰
□	area 6	posterior sector of the superior, middle and inferior frontal gyri; premotor region; the mesial surface = supplementary motor area
⊡	area 10	⎫
″	area 9	superior and middle frontal gyri; dorsolateral and mesial prefrontal region;
★	area 8	⎭
∩	area 46	middle frontal gyrus; dorsolateral prefrontal region;
✕	area 32	mesial superior frontal gyrus;
⊙	area 11,12	orbital gyri;
⊚	area 25	subcallosal area; limbic cortex
●	area 24	anterior cingulate gyrus; limbic cortex
S	area 3,1,2	postcentral gyrus; primary sensory cortices
¦	area 40	supramarginal gyrus; ⎱ inferior parietal lobule
v	area 39	angular gyrus; ⎰
▲	area 7	superior parietal lobule;
⊘	area 5	anterosuperior sector of superior parietal lobule;
O	area 23,31	posterior half of cingulate gyrus; limbic cortex
◕	area 30,26,29	retrosplenial area; limbic cortex
T	area 22	superior (first) temporal gyrus; auditory association cortex; left posterior third = Wernicke area
⋙	area 41,42	transverse gyri of Heschl; primary auditory cortex
◪	area 21	middle (second) temporal gyrus;
·/	area 20	inferior (third) temporal gyrus;
∴	area 35,36	fourth temporal gyrus;
Ŧ	area 37	posterior sector of middle, inferior and fourth temporal gyri;
━●━	area 28,27	parahippocampal (fifth temporal) gyrus; limbic cortex
⚮	area 38	temporal pole; limbic cortex
x	area 17	calcarine region; primary visual cortex
▲	area 18	lingual and fusiform gyri below the calcarine region; precuneus above the calcarine region; visual association cortices
--	area 19	

Association cortex groupings (right brace annotations):
- areas 10, 9, 8, 46, 32, 11,12 = association cortex
- areas 40, 39, 7, 5 = association cortex
- areas 21, 20, 35,36, 37 = association cortex

THEMATIC INDEX OF ILLUSTRATIONS

LANGUAGE AND SPEECH DISORDERS

Broca's Aphasia   Figures 2.19–2.21; 4.4
Wernicke's Aphasia   Figures 3.1; 3.17; 3.22; 3.23A; 3.26
Conduction Aphasia   Figures 2.16; 4.7
Global Aphasia   Figures 2.17–2.19; 4.21–4.22
Transcortical Motor Aphasia   Figures 4.11–4.12
Transcortical Sensory Aphasia   Figure 2.15
Basal Ganglia Aphasia   Figure 2.14
Thalamic Aphasia   Figure 2.15; 3.25
Akinetic Mutism   Figure 2.22
Anomia   Figures 3.26; 3.27

VISUAL DISORDERS

Achromatopsia   Figures 2.6; 2.8
Visual Field Defect Without Achromatopsia   Figures 2.7; 4.18–4.19
Alexia Without Agraphia   Figures 2.6; 3.12
Prosopagnosia   Figures 2.8; 3.6A–3.7A
Simultanagnosia   Figure 2.9
Optic Ataxia   Figure 2.10
Neglect   Figures 2.12; 3.28–3.29

MEMORY DISORDERS

Global Amnesic Syndromes   Figures 2.13; 3.6B–3.7B; 3.13–3.14
Amnesia in Degenerative Dementias   Figures 3.2–3.3; 3.8–3.11
Anosognosia   Figures 2.11–2.12; 3.28–3.29

ACQUIRED PERSONALITY DISORDERS   Figure 2.11

TYPES OF PATHOLOGY

Non-hemorrhagic Infarctions   Figures 2.6–2.10; 2.12; 2.14–2.15; 2.17–2.22; 3.6–3.7; 3.12; 3.17; 3.24–3.30; 4.4; 4.7; 4.9; 4.11–4.12; 4.14–4.15; 4.18–4.22

Hemorrhagic Infarctions and Intracerebral Hematomas   Figures 3.22; 3.23

Herpes Simplex Encephalitis   Figures 2.13; 3.13–3.14

Tumors   Figures 2.11; 3.15–3.16; 3.21

Surgical Ablations   Figures 2.11; 2.16; 3.18–3.21

Degenerative Diseases   Figures 3.2–3.3; 3.8–3.11

TECHNICAL ASPECTS OF INTERPRETATION

Timing of CT   Figures 3.1; 3.24–3.25; 3.28; 3.30

Charting of Lesions in CT and MR   Figures 4.4–4.6; 4.8–4.15; 4.21–4.22

Charting of Abnormalities in SPET   Figures 3.4–3.5

Pathologic Confirmation of CT Images   Figures 2.9; 3.12

INDEX